MEDICAL PRACTICE MANAGEMENT
Body of Knowledge Review

3.5 Edition

FINANCIAL MANAGEMENT

VOLUME 2

MGMA
104 Inverness Terrace East
Englewood, CO 80112-5306
877.275.6462
mgma.com

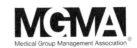

MGMA

Medical Group Management Association®

Body of Knowledge Review Series - Edition 3.5

VOLUME 1: Operations Management

VOLUME 2: Financial Management

VOLUME 3: Human Resource Management

VOLUME 4: Organizational Governance and
Patient-Centered Care

VOLUME 5: Risk and Compliance Management

Library of Congress Cataloging-in-Publication Data

Names: MGMA (Association), issuing body.
Title: Financial management.
Other titles: Financial management (Medical Group Management Association) | Medical practice management body of knowledge review (3.5 edition) ; v. 2.
Description: Englewood, CO : MGMA, [2019] | Series: Medical practice management body of knowledge review (3.5 edition) ; volume 2 | Includes bibliographical references and index.
Identifiers: LCCN 2019047346 (print) | LCCN 2019047347 (ebook) | ISBN 9781568296937 (paperback) | ISBN 9781568296944 (ebook)
Subjects: MESH: Financial Management--organization & administration | Practice Management, Medical--economics
Classification: LCC R728 (print) | LCC R728 (ebook) | NLM W 80 | DDC 610.68/1--dc23
LC record available at https://lccn.loc.gov/2019047346
LC ebook record available at https://lccn.loc.gov/2019047347

Item: 1026
ISBN: 978-1-56829-693-7

Printed in the United States of America

10 9 8 7 6 5 4 3 2 1

Contents

Introduction

Financial management is the cornerstone of every medical practice. And while many of the same competencies are required for managers in any organization, there are particular nuances specific to the delivery of healthcare in a clinic setting that differentiate the medical practice administrator from his or her peers in other business or healthcare delivery environments. The chapters in this volume follow the blueprint designed by practicing medical practice executives to describe the key competencies, knowledge, and skills required to develop and maintain the financial well-being of the medical practice.

The major areas of competence, as identified by the Medical Group Management Association (MGMA) members, required for effective financial management of a medical practice are to:

- Develop, implement, and manage the revenue cycle;
- Manage cash flow;
- Manage accounts payable;
- Manage payroll;
- Create and manage budgets; and
- Manage the audit process.

Within each chapter of this volume, these major competencies are further delineated according to the key knowledge and skills required to demonstrate competency as a financial manager. A few examples of these supporting skills are the ability to develop and implement internal financial controls, the knowledge to build and analyze key financial documents, the skill to manage cash transactions, and the ability to manage payer contracts. These knowledge and skills and many others are explored in detail in the pages that follow.

Chapter 1

Understanding the Revenue Cycle

In most industries, when a business sends a bill, it expects that the customer will pay 100 percent of the amount billed. This is not the case for much of the healthcare industry, and understanding your practice's revenue cycle can have a tremendous effect on its bottom line. The billing and collection process is complex, with multiple payers, varying fee schedules, numerous rules and regulations, compliance challenges, and many opportunities for practices to fail to receive payment for services.

Medical practices normally bill numerous insurance companies and government payers, each of whom reimburses the practice according to its own negotiated or government mandated fee schedules. Those fee schedules contain contractual allowances, or discounts, off the practice's stated fee schedule. Further complicating this process, some patients are insured by more than one payer. The practice must submit bills (or claims) to the payers in a standardized format, in compliance with government regulations and payer policies. Payers may refuse to pay some of the claims for various reasons, such as incomplete or incorrect information, late filing, or claims that the services were "not medically necessary."

On some occasions, the practice does not receive a reply to a claim from the payer and must follow up. In response, the payer may indicate that it never received the claim or provide other excuses for nonpayment. Practice managers need to ensure that their billing department staff or billing company works on denials and past due claims to get paid for its services. Insured patients are often liable for portions of their bills in the form of copayments, coinsurances, or deductibles. A growing number of uninsured patients and higher deductible health plans have resulted in practices needing to collect more of their fees from patients. Although collecting from insurance companies can present challenges, patients often have financial problems or conflicting priorities that also make collecting fees difficult.

The key skills and knowledge necessary to successfully manage the financial health of a medical practice include:

- Managing front-end operations, including scheduling, insurance verification, authorizations, copayments, and deductibles collection;
- Overseeing medical record documentation, charge capture, and coding;
- Managing charge audit;
- Submitting claims and resolving edits;
- Implementing accounts receivable follow-up and refund processes;
- Monitoring and reporting key metrics;
- Analyzing reimbursement and reviewing contracts;
- Managing and negotiating payer contracts;
- Managing charge masters and payment schedules; and
- Managing payer credentialing.

Coding and Charge Capture

Coding

Every code that is billed should be adequately documented by the physician in the medical records. In the eyes of the Office of Inspector General, U.S. Department of Health and Human Services, if a service wasn't documented, it wasn't performed. Practices should keep current coding publications on hand to assist the coders in complying with applicable laws and regulations. Having both internal and external audits helps facilitate compliance. The physicians are ultimately responsible for coding.

The practice must include both a procedure code using Current Procedural Terminology (CPT®)* and at least one corresponding diagnosis code using *International Classification of Diseases, 10th revision, Clinical Modification* (ICD-10-CM), to get paid by third-party payers. In addition to the basic CPT code, the practice may need to add one or more modifiers to better describe the service. For example, the modifier "26" signifies the professional (provider) component.[1]

Although Medicare generally requires use of CPT codes, regional carriers may require use of the Healthcare Common Procedure Coding System (HCPCS) for certain services, such as durable medical equipment, flu injections, and screening Pap smears.

The practice needs to ensure that the codes accurately describe the services provided and the related diagnosis. Common coding compliance issues include the National Correct Coding Initiative (NCCI) and selecting the correct evaluation and management code for office visits, consultations, and other cognitive services provided by the physicians.

National Correct Coding Initiative

The Centers for Medicare & Medicaid Services (CMS) implemented the NCCI in 1996.[2] This program aims to control Medicare costs by identifying improper coding on claims and denying reimbursement for those claims.

For example, a practice may bill multiple codes for service that CMS believes should have been combined or "bundled" as one code. Other edits may deny a particular code when it is billed with a code that CMS holds to be incompatible. The Medically Unlikely Edits (MUEs) deny units of service for a CPT or HCPCS code that exceed the number

---

* CPT © 2015 American Medical Association. All rights reserved.

considered to be the maximum units of that service provided to a single beneficiary on a single day of service.

Practices need to ensure compliance with correct coding rules. A practice may override some of those edits by using a modifier that indicates that the edit should not apply in this circumstance. Practices need to ensure that they use those overriding modifiers only when appropriate. The practice will file its claims with the appropriate organization (or "carrier") in its area.

Charge Capture

The practice should implement policies and procedures to ensure that it accurately bills all services performed. Some practices adopting electronic health records (EHRs) report improved charge capture by doing so.

Many practices capture office charges using prenumbered patient encounter forms. The physicians complete that form during or shortly after the patient encounter. The form should provide space for the physician to indicate the procedure(s) performed, level of service, and related diagnosis. The form can also be used to track laboratory orders and provide receipts for patients.

Capturing services performed in a hospital or other outside setting, such as a nursing home, can be difficult for an office-based practice. Business office personnel and medical office staff are generally not present at these remote locations to register the patient and handle the related paperwork at the time of service.

Practices also find that they sometimes neglect billing for all ancillary services, drugs, and supplies. Failure to document a service means not being able to bill for that service. Failure to bill a service means a zero chance of collecting for that service.

Hospital-Based Physician Charge Capture

Some hospital-based groups capture their hospital charges, including the procedure and diagnosis codes, via an interface between the hospital data system and the practice data system. Other hospital-based practices continue to rely on paper copies of the charge data. Those practices should ensure that they have captured all charges by accounting for all of the accession numbers from the hospital.

Billing software packages can often produce a "missing number" report to expedite locating the missing charges. In addition to capturing charge data, hospital-based practices must often capture the related demographic information through an interface between the two systems.

Understanding Payer Types

Unlike most businesses that only accept payments from customers or other businesses, medical practices collect money from a variety of payers. These include commercial payers, the government, workers' compensation, and the patients themselves. You must understand all of them to maximize collections and boost net revenue.

Commercial Payers

In 1850, the Franklin Health Assurance Company of Massachusetts offered insurance coverage for medical expenses.[3] Other private insurance companies also developed plans that reimbursed patients for their healthcare expenditures. In 1943, tax laws allowed corporations to deduct the cost of healthcare for their employees.[4] Furthermore, those costs were not considered part of the employees' wages. This provided a mechanism for corporations to legally provide additional compensation to their employees without violating World War II wage controls.

Employer-provided health insurance expanded rapidly, beginning a shift in the cost of healthcare from the individual to the employer. Today, Blue Cross Blue Shield is our nation's largest provider of health benefits, with 36 companies nationwide and customers in all 50 states, Blue Cross Blue Shield insures nearly one in three Americans. More than 95 percent of U.S. physicians contract with a Blue Cross Blue Shield carrier.[5]

Many specialties report that their charges for commercial patients represent a significantly lower percentage of their payer mix. This is likely because the population covered by commercial insurance is younger and requires fewer health services than the population covered by Medicare. For example, internal medicine, cardiology, ophthalmology, and urology report that fewer than half of their patients had commercial insurance.

Patients with commercial insurance accounted for less than 60 percent of the patient mix for gastroenterology, neurology, anesthesiology, orthopedic surgery, and general surgery practices. Pediatrics and OB/GYN, which have a younger patient base, reported the highest level of commercial patients.

Managed Care

Physicians historically had considerable autonomy over treatment options and the amount they charged for their services. Beginning in the 1980s, health insurance companies responded to rapidly increasing medical costs and insurance use by taking steps to control costs.[6] Health plans began negotiating with physicians to accept discounted fee schedules. Those payers also instituted policies to "manage" the manner in which physicians and other providers practice medicine. New types of commercial health plans appeared on the market. The methods that those organizations use to manage care include:

- Requiring that certain surgeries be performed on an outpatient basis;
- Performing same-day admission surgery;
- Using drug formularies;
- Limiting the number of times that insurance will pay for a particular procedure during a set time;
- Requiring advance approval for certain procedures and medications;
- Requiring referrals as a prerequisite for reimbursing many procedures performed by specialists; and
- Reviewing charges to determine medical necessity.

More aggressive managed care models involve capitation and assumption of financial risk by the practice. Capitation and discounted fee-for-service will be discussed in the section on payment methods. Following are two of the more popular forms of managed care plans.

- **Health maintenance organizations (HMOs):** An HMO is a healthcare system that assumes or shares both the financial risks and the delivery risks associated with providing comprehensive medical services to a voluntarily enrolled population in a particular geographic area, usually in return for a fixed, prepaid fee.
- **Preferred provider organizations (PPOs):** A PPO is a medical plan in which coverage is provided to participants through a network of selected healthcare providers (such as hospitals and physicians). The enrollees may go outside the network, but they would pay a greater percentage of the cost of coverage than within the network
- **Health exchange plans:** Health exchange plans (also known as marketplace plans or "Obamacare plans") began operating in all states on October 1, 2013, as required by the Patient Protection and Accountable Care Act (ACA) as a mechanism to provide coverage for individuals who did not otherwise have access to coverage. These plans cannot exclude coverage for preexisting conditions and must provide a basic benefit package that includes preventive care as well as catastrophic coverage. Government subsidies are available to those meeting certain income limitations. These plans often use cost management tactics similar to those used by HMOs and PPOs.

Private Pay and Self-Pay

Uninsured patients are not the only individuals from whom practices must collect money. Insured patients are often responsible for a portion of their medical bills, as most government and commercial plans include some element of patient responsibility. High-deductible health plans, sometimes combined with health savings accounts (HSAs), are increasing in popularity.

HSAs are tax-advantaged savings accounts that allow individuals to set aside money for future medical, retirement, or long-term care premium expenses. Only participants enrolled in a qualified high deductible health plan are eligible for these plans. The balances can be rolled over from year to year, and participants can take them with them when they change jobs.

Government Payers

Although employer health plans grew rapidly during the years following World War II, elderly people were often retired and thus not eligible for the coverage. Because insurance companies often rated their premiums based on claims history, individual coverage for the elderly was often quite expensive.

Although a presidential committee had considered government health coverage for senior citizens as early as 1934, this did not become a reality until 1965, when President Lyndon Johnson signed an amended Social Security Act. This act created Medicare for most Americans older than age 65 (those receiving benefits from Social Security or the Railroad Retirement Board) and Medicaid for some of the indigent. Those younger than 65 who had long-term disabilities or end stage renal disease joined the list of eligible Medicare recipients in 1972.[7]

Medicare

Medicare Part B was created as a separate plan to provide physician compensation. Approximately 99 percent of Medicare patients have worked at least 40 quarters of Medicare covered employment and thus do not pay for Part A (facility care). Almost all Medicare participants elect Part B coverage.

Medicare Advantage Programs

Earlier, we discussed the fact that commercial payers became concerned about increasing healthcare costs and began managed care initiatives to try to control escalating healthcare costs. Controlling government spending for healthcare became a concern as well. The Tax Equity and Fiscal Responsibility Act (1982) made contracting with Medicare easier for HMOs.

In an attempt to privatize some aspects of Medicare, Medicare Advantage, and Medicare+Choice plans were introduced in 1997.[8] Medicare Advantage plans may be offered in HMO, PPO, private fee-for-service, or special needs plans. The practice and its physicians need to contract separately with these plans. Some of these plans reimburse at Medicare rates, while others have their own fee schedule.

Medicaid

Medicaid funding was available to the states beginning Jan. 1, 1966,[9] and was phased in by the states, which administer the program, over several years.

The focus of Medicaid is to cover children and pregnant women living near or below the poverty level. It is not surprising that Medical Group Management Association® (MGMA®) survey data report the highest percentages of Medicaid patients in pediatric and OB/GYN practices.

Other Government Payers

One such government payer is TRICARE for military healthcare. It was formerly known as the Civilian Health and Medical Program of the Uniformed Services. Another payer is the Civilian Health and Medical Program of the Department of Veterans Affairs.

Workers' Compensation

Most employers must purchase workers' compensation insurance to compensate employees for on-the-job injuries and pay the related medical bills. As both employers and providers of medical services, physician practices often find that they purchase the insurance for their employees and also bill for the relevant services provided by patients.

For most specialties, workers' compensation constitutes a very small portion of their gross charges. A notable exception is orthopedic surgery. The regulations for billing and reimbursement by workers' compensation vary by state. Practice managers must be familiar with the applicable state's regulations in order to maximize workers' compensation reimbursement.

Methods of Reimbursement and Payment Models

Getting paid presents special challenges for physician practices, whether it is collecting from the patient or a third-party payer. The practice administrator and the billing staff need to be familiar with the various methods that third-party payers use to pay providers. Practice personnel must figure out a process to collect from patients who are now responsible for an increasing portion of their bills. As previously discussed, this is because of the increasing number of uninsured patients, as well as the increasing popularity of high-deductible health insurance plans and HSAs.

Traditional Fee-for-Service

Historically, physicians have been paid on a fee-for-service basis. In the past, most health insurance policies were indemnity policies. Patients visited the physician of their choice and paid the physician. The insurance company would reimburse the patient for the amount of the physician's charges less any patient responsibility for deductibles or coinsurance. The payment would be reduced if the physicians' billed charge exceeded the amount the insurance company determined to be usual and customary. The physician would collect his or her fee from the patient in this situation.

If physicians accepted assignment for their services, they would bill the insurance company on their patients' behalf and the insurance company would pay the physicians. Physicians could then bill patients for any patient due balance or collect at the time of the service.

Under traditional fee-for-service, physicians had the freedom to set their fees and collect (or attempt to collect) those fees in full from the patients and their insurance companies. Patients had the freedom to choose their physicians. Indemnity arrangements still exist today but are not common and are decreasing in popularity.

Discounted Fee-for-Service

Beginning with the advent of managed care in the 1980s, the most common method commercial payers used to control costs was to negotiate with providers, who agreed to be paid a discount off their usual fee in exchange for being a participating provider with that payer. As participating providers, physicians had the benefit of *steerage*, meaning that the payer provided financial incentives for the patients to use participating physicians.

Resource-Based Relative Value System

Initially, Medicare reimbursement was based on charges, which was the same method that commercial insurers used at the time. Although Medicare put limits on reimbursement in an early attempt to control costs, physicians could bill patients for any amount that Medicare did not pay. In 1992, Medicare implemented a fee schedule determining the amount doctors could collect for services to Medicare patients.[10] This fee schedule was based on a comprehensive study of the relative cost of the resources used (including malpractice, practice expense, and work of the provider) to provide each medical service a value as compared to other services. This was called the *resource-based relative value system* (RBRVS).

The RBRVS assigns relative values to most of the CPT codes. The values are based on the resources that a physician typically uses to perform the service. The resources are divided into three parts:

1. Physician work — time, technical skill, physical strength, mental effort and judgment, physician stress, and total work;

2. Practice expenses — rent, support staff, supplies, and other items that may vary with the physician's gross revenue, mix of services, and practice location; and

3. Malpractice expenses — costs that vary by specialty.

The RBRVS uses relative values — nonmonetary, relative units of measure — for most of the CPT (CPT-4) codes. It converts these relative values into dollar amounts by applying a conversion factor. The Medicare program uses a single conversion factor that it updates annually in the Medicare fee schedule. Then a geographic component adjusts the payments according to regional differences in the cost of living and physician practice costs. Private insurance carriers tend to use different conversion factors.

Although the RBRVS was developed as a reimbursement mechanism, the data can be used in other ways. Because relative value units (RVUs) summarize the relative weight of procedures performed by physicians for all patients, regardless of the payer or the physician's charges, administrators can use them to evaluate how much an individual physician's activities contribute to practice profits. Administrators can also use RVUs to estimate the cost of services provided or determine a physician's compensation.

To develop its own RVUs, a practice can extract procedure code data from its billing system and relate those data to the relative value weights for each procedure as assigned by the Medicare RBRVS. The RVUs are calculated as follows:

> **Total Relative Value Units =**
> **Total Procedures Performed × Value Units**

The relative values are multiplied by a conversion factor to calculate the fee schedule amount for each service. Initially, the RBRVS was designed to be budget neutral. The related study indicated that the fees Medicare had been paying for surgery and other complex procedures were high in relation to those for office visits and consultations. Consequently, RBRVS increased payments to general practitioners while reducing amounts paid to specialists. Although the initial fee schedule was budget neutral, the conversion schedule was to be updated annually for changes in physicians' costs and also to counteract changes in the volume of services per beneficiary.

When the RBRVS was introduced, many predicted that commercial payers would adopt the fee schedule Medicare created. Some have done this, while others have created their own fee schedule based on RBRVS data.

Today the RBRVS and RVUs have uses beyond the fee schedule. Practices use them to measure physician productivity, allocate costs, assign staff, and determine cost per procedure. Medicaid and workers' compensation are controlled by the states. Those payers have their own fee schedules which limit the amount that physicians can collect for services to those patients.

Contractual Allowances

Because of the large volume of business with Medicare and other governmental payers that require discounted fee schedules and discounted fee-for-service contracts with commercial payers, today's medical practices find that they do a considerable amount of business at lower rates than their billed charges. Because they are forbidden either by contract or by law to collect the difference, practices must write off the difference between their billed charge and the contracted reimbursement. The write-offs are called *contractual allowances*. Be aware that even if a practice does not participate with some government payers, it is often restricted in the amount that it can collect from those patients.

Silent Preferred Provider Organizations

Silent PPOs are payers that attempt to obtain discounts similar to contractual allowances without providing a contractual obligation to the provider. Some of those payers promote themselves as legitimate PPOs. Sometimes they falsely claim a discount from another network in which the provider does participate. Practices should consider whether or not to accept a discounted fee they are not legally required to accept when the payer has not provided any steerage or incentive for patients to use the practice.

Capitation

One payment method that some managed care organizations use to reimburse for services is *capitation* or prepaid services. Under this model, the payer and the provider negotiate a fixed periodic payment (usually monthly) paid to the provider to provide specific healthcare services to an attributed patient population. Those payments are often quoted in terms of *per member per month.* Because services and utilization vary by patient age and sex, it is important to have demographic information regarding the covered population when determining the appropriate rate.

The manner in which the practice becomes profitable differs significantly between capitation and fee-for-service. Under fee-for-service, higher volumes of services generally result in higher levels of profit. Under capitation, the practice is paid whether it sees the patients or not; consequently, lower volumes of services are more profitable; higher volume results in higher variable costs, such as medical supplies, laundry and linens, drugs, postage, and some billing costs.

Even though volume under a capitated contract does not affect the amount of payment, the practice will still need to file a claim with the payer. The payers need a detailed record of the services performed for their patients in order to manage the insured population.

Under advanced forms of capitation, providers assume financial risk for the patient population. This is sometimes referred to as *global capitation.* The provider group's reimbursement includes payment for the total delivery of healthcare services within a specified scope. Depending on the services, these contracts can be full or shared risk. For example, a group of primary care physicians or a multispecialty clinic may provide most services under a risk contract and assume responsibility for paying outside specialists to whom they refer those patients

Value-Based Care

Value-based care, also known as pay for performance, or P4P, ties physician payments and other healthcare provider payments to defined medical standards. The movement began as a way to improve quality in the healthcare system by holding providers financially accountable for their services.

In 2007, Medicare initiated its initial version of value-based care, the Physician Quality Reporting System (PQRS).[12] The program rewarded or punished physicians with a positive, neutral or negative adjustment to their Medicare payments based upon their reporting of certain quality measures. The Medicare Access and CHIP Reauthorization Act of 2015 (MACRA) created a more comprehensive program that increased the reporting requirements, the types of providers included, and the related risk/reward.

Providers can participate in MACRA either as a member of an Advanced Alternative Payment Model (APM) or using the Merit-based Incentive System (MIPS). Advanced APMs operate as either:

- A Medical Home Model under CMS Innovation Center Authority; or
- Require members to assume significant financial risk.

Providers participating in an Advanced APM may potentially receive a 5 percent bonus and are exempt from MIPS.

Eligible providers (those who are eligible clinician types and meet certain minimum volume thresholds) who do not participate in an Advanced APM are included in MIPS. For MIPS, providers report under four categories:

1. **Quality** *(This replaced the former PQRS discussed above.)*

2. **Promoting Interoperability** *(This replaced the Medicare EHR Incentive Program, also known as Meaningful Use.)*

3. **Improvement Activities** *(For this new category, participants self-report from an inventory of activities that improve the care process, patient engagement and/or access to care.)*

4. **Cost** *(This is calculated by CMS based upon claims.)*

Some providers will not report in all categories. For example, providers who are nonpatient facing (as determined by CMS) are not required to report in the Promoting Interoperability category. Also, CMS does not report a cost component for all providers. Scores for providers reporting in less than four categories are reweighted[1]

MIPS is designed to be budget neutral, with providers receiving positive, negative or neutral adjustments to their Medicare payments based upon their MIPS reporting, as follows:

MIPS Reporting Year	Medicare Payment Adjustment Year	Adjustment Range
2017	2019	+/ 4%
2018	2020	+/ 5%
2019	2021	+/ 7%
2020	2022	+/ 9%

Private payers may also have quality reporting programs. These take several common forms. For example, a typical program will reward a physician with a bonus depending on how well he or she performs on certain quality measures and/or may use the Healthcare Effectiveness Data and Information Set (HEDIS) standards to rate the physician or provider, according to the National Committee for Quality Assurance (NCQA).

If a practice elects to participate in a quality care program, it will need to ensure that it provides all the necessary information to the payer.

Third-Party Payers

When a practice files a claim with a third-party payer, it should receive an *explanation of benefits* (EOB) or *electronic remittance advice* (ERA) form from the payer within the time stipulated in the contract or by state law. The form may be accompanied by a check in payment of its services if the funds are not electronically remitted. The EOB explains how the payer computed the amount it paid (or did not pay) for the claim. This information is generally itemized by CPT code or description and includes the:

- Gross amount of claim;
- Amount allowable;
- Amount excluded and reason it was excluded;
- Amount of patient responsibility and explanation (i.e., copayment, deductible, or coinsurance); and
- Amount paid or denial of the claim with the reason for the denial.

The following discussion about posting the payment and handling the other information on the EOB assumes the practice handles its own billing. If the practice outsources its billing, then the billing company will perform these functions.

First, the payment poster should ensure that contractual allowances and allowable amounts on the EOB are correct according to the practice's contract. If a check accompanies the EOB, the payment amount should be posted to the patient's account along with any contractual write off. Most practice management systems allow the practice to enter its fee schedules by payer into the system; the system should alert the poster to any incorrect amounts. (The practice needs to ensure that the fee schedules in its system are current or this tool will not be effective.) If the contractual allowance or payment is incorrect, a staff member should be responsible for following up on errors. Failure to write off a contractual allowance for a payer with whom the practice participates is a violation of the practice's contract with that payer.

The practice should audit or review the work done by its payment posters on a regular basis to ensure that they are handling the contractual allowances properly. For example, if staff members write off patient responsibility or adjustments made by payers with whom the practice does not participate, the practice loses that money.

If there is a remaining patient due balance after posting the payment, a bill should be sent to the patient. The sooner the practice sends it, the sooner the practice will be paid.

Third-Party Reimbursement

The bulk of accounts receivable (A/R) funds due to most practices is from insurance companies and government payers. For accounting purposes, it is important to differentiate between charges (practice fees), allowables (amount to be collected by contract from the insurance company and patient), and paid amount (what the insurance company and patient pays).

Payer payments come to the practice with an EOB. Patient payments are generally in the form of copayments collected at the time of service and deductibles paid after billing patients for their portion of the outstanding balance. Ideally, the combined insurance and patient payment will equal the allowable, which will equal what the contract says should be paid. It is important that the practice knows what the contractual allowable should be to avoid underpayments.

Contractual allowables are based on each payer's contract and, in some cases, the provider manual or other documents referenced in the contract. Some practices calculate the allowable amount due for their more common services and compare the payer's EOB statement to this list. Other practices have the entire allowable schedule for all services built into their practice system for automated comparisons. This claim-by-claim audit reduces the possibility of underpayment.

Denial Management

Denial management relates to the nonpayment of claims (the practice bill) by insurance companies. The effective management of denials is one of the more complex parts of overall A/R collections, but it is necessary to avoid potentially significant cumulative losses over time. As with most complex problems, it is best to break denial management into small parts.

The first step is to review the EOBs and categorize the reasons for denials given by insurance companies. Examples include "not a benefit," "no referral," "patient not insured," "service not matching age/sex/ diagnosis of the patient," "service not covered under patient's contract,"

18

and many others. Payers have a long list of denial codes, and these are usually identified on the EOB. Medicare and most commercial payers use the standard set of Claim Adjustment Reason Codes (CARC) used to describe the denial, as well as Remittance Advice Remark Codes (RARC), which provide additional information about the adjustment. The standard code set is available from The Washington Publishing Company website. A practice should develop its own list of the most frequently used denial codes so that payer codes can easily be aggregated for statistical purposes. Payers can then be benchmarked against each other to determine trends and patterns.

The practice's denial codes should be broad enough to segregate denials caused by practice coding issues and those that are payer driven. Every effort should be made to identify and correct internal causes of denials. Reducing denials not only improves cash flow, it decreases rework expenses related to claims processing.

Inappropriate payer denials should be managed aggressively. Correcting (if necessary) and resubmitting the denied claim will rectify the majority of problems for most payers. If this does not work, then the next step is to appeal the denial in accordance with the payer's process. The appeal should be tracked and followed until it is resolved. If there are a large number of similar denials from the same payer, senior payer management should address the issue so that the payer's claims processing system is corrected. Before these issues escalate into a major confrontation, make sure the issue is large enough in terms of total dollars to warrant the extra effort.

Finally, the payer/practice contract or state regulations may require payers to meet certain standards on claim reimbursement to avoid paying penalties or interest. Be aware of these requirements and make sure you collect what is due. If the state requires interest to be paid and the payer does not pay it, consider asking the state insurance commissioner for assistance.

Administrative Follow-up for Denials

If the payer denies all or part of a claim, the reasons for the denial should be included on the EOB or ERA. Denials may be attributable to practice errors or oversight when submitting the claim or they might be due to payer errors.

The practice should assign responsibility for following up on denials to the billing staff. Insurance follow-up staff or the payment posters may perform the function.

Tracking errors that occur frequently, such as claims filed with the wrong modifier, can often indicate a systemic problem in the practice's billing process. If the practice can correct the problem, it will reduce its denials in the future (and collect money faster). If a payer is denying claims inappropriately, the practice needs to address the problem with the payer by meeting with the payer representative.

The practice should also maintain a file of documentation regarding problems with individual payers. It can be useful as a reference when renegotiating a payer contract. Ensure that denials are noted on the patient's financial account notes, even when the claim does not include a payment. The documentation will assist the insurance follow-up staff in taking appropriate action on a claim. All of the office staff should be able to determine the process steps and explain the account status to patients and the payers based on the notes.

Follow-up

Designated billing personnel need to follow up on unpaid claims within a specified time period as part of their normal responsibilities. Common reasons that the practice may have unpaid claims include:

- The payer maintains the claim was not received;
- The payer claims the EOB or check was mailed but the practice never received it;
- The payer may have mailed the payment to the patient; and

- The payer may be waiting on more information from other providers or payers before the claim is adjudicated.

Withhold Tracking

Withholds occur when the payer retains part of the payment for a period of time, to be returned at a later date if certain payer and provider objectives are met. This mainly applies to capitation payments, but not fee-for-service. In general, it is not a good contracting policy to let someone else hold the practice's money with a promise to pay at some indefinite time and under vague parameters. Unfortunately, the repayment of withholds to practices isn't as common as the collection of withholds by payers.

If withholds cannot be avoided, the practice should track how much has been withheld over the period of time and follow up with requests for payment. Some practices book the withhold due as an account receivable until reconciled. Exercise due diligence. It helps to periodically reconcile with the payer how much is in the withhold account so that disputes are avoided at the end of the withhold period. The basis on which the withhold is repaid or not repaid should be examined and audited if necessary.

Monitoring the Audit Trail

When practices submit claims electronically, transmission and acceptance reports will create an audit trail indicating which claims were successfully transmitted and received by the payer and which were not. These reports from your clearinghouse are known as EDI 276/277 transaction set. Practices need to ensure that a billing staff person is responsible for monitoring these reports and correcting claims that did not process or transmit correctly. The faster those are corrected, the faster the practice can get paid.

Transmission and acceptance reports provide confirmation that claims were filed and received, unlike filing paper claims by mail. It is better to know immediately that claims did not process properly than to discover them 30 days later when the claim shows up in the aged insurance follow-up queue.

Financial Responsibility

Commercial and government payers often do not pay the entire allowable fee. The patient must frequently bear a portion of the cost in the form of a copayment, coinsurance, or deductible.

Exhibit 1.1 provides various patient responsibility amounts and Exhibit 1.2 illustrates how a patient's responsibility for a copayment, deductible, or coinsurance amount interacts with the third-party payer's obligation to pay for covered services.

Secondary Insurance Coverage

Some patients are covered by more than one payer. For example, a patient may be covered by a policy sponsored by her own employer and another sponsored by her husband's employer. A person who has reached age 65 and is still working may be covered by both his employer's health plan and Medicare.

When a patient has two insurance policies, one is the primary insurance and the other is secondary. For example, the employer's plan is often, but not always, primary for a person who is covered by both his or her employer's plan and Medicare. Assuming the commercial policy is primary, Medicare would be the secondary payer in this case. Determining which insurance is primary and which is secondary can be confusing, and sometimes the payers even disagree.

The practice should bill the primary insurance first. After the primary insurance has paid or settled, the practice should then bill the secondary insurance. Medicare will automatically bill the secondary insurance (called) for most plans. After the practice has settled the claim with the secondary insurer, the practice may then bill the patient if there is a patient-due portion remaining.

This process, called *coordination of benefits*, often takes longer than collecting from a patient who has only one insurance policy. Consequently, payers may have longer filing deadlines for submitting claims to the secondary insurance.

Exhibit 1.1		
Definitions of Patient Responsibility Amounts		
Type of Patient Responsibility	**Description**	**Example**
Copayments	Revenues generated from payment-sharing arrangements between the insurance carrier or federal entity and the patient, which often includes the concept of a specific amount of money per visit	Contract requires patient to pay $25 per office visit
Coinsurance	The percentage of allowable charges that patients insured by a third-party payer are required to pay according to their contract with the third-party payer	Contract requires that patient be responsible for 20% of allowable charges
Deductible	Amount of allowable charges that a patient covered by a third-party payer is required to pay out of pocket before the payer begins reimbursing for covered services	The Part B Medicare deductible is $185 for 2019; thus patients must pay $185 of allowable costs for calendar year 2019 before Medicare begins paying for these services
Noncovered charge	A charge that the payer will not pay; the practice should check its contract to ensure that it can collect from the patient for this service; a waiver or other type of notice (such as an Advance Beneficiary Notice of Noncoverage [ABN]) may be required	A contract may not cover cosmetic surgery but permit the provider to bill the patient for this service

Profiling Payers

Much has been written about payers profiling or rating physicians based on quality and cost of services. It is recommended that the practice keep track of payer performance. This type of information can be valuable when renegotiating the contract. A payer that creates chaos in the billing office should pay a higher contract rate than the payer who

Exhibit 1.2

Collecting Discounted Fee-for-Service with Copayments, Coinsurance, and Deductibles

Assumptions:

- Practice is a participating provider with the third-party payer
- Gross charge $125
- Contractual write-off $25
- Copayments, coinsurance, deductibles as per the individual examples

Example 1: Patient has a $15 copayment.

Gross Charge $125		
Allowable Amount $100		
Third-party payer pays $85 allowable amount less Copayment: $85	Patient responsible for the $15 copayment.	Contractual write off (the practice cannot collect this amount): $25

Example 2: Patient owes 20% coinsurance.

Gross Charge $125		
Allowable Amount $100		
Third-party payer pays 80% of the allowable amount: $80.	Patient responsible for the 20% coinsurance: $20.	Contractual write off (the practice cannot collect this amount): $25

Example 3: Patient has a $15 copayment, plus a $500 deductible (not yet met), $85 of which is applied to this service.

Gross Charge $125		
Allowable Amount $100		
Patient is responsible for the rest of the allowable amount because the deductible has not yet been met: $85.	Patient responsible for the $15 copayment.	Contractual write off (the practice cannot collect this amount): $25

pays accurately and on time. Variables that should be tracked include claims payment accuracy and timeliness, number and type of denials, resolution of appeals and other problems, and contract negotiations. The list should be comprehensive enough to evaluate a payer's performance fairly against other payers.

Auditing Payments

Managing the individual claim EOBs is only one way to improve collections. Having an internal audit program to supplement EOB processing is another. The goal in auditing the payer is to determine whether or not the practice is being paid correctly and the payer is complying with the terms of the contract.

There are four steps to consider when structuring the auditing process for the practice. They are:

1. Organize your contract files;
2. Identify and monitor key indicators from the contract;
3. Track and document discrepancies; and
4. Prepare to mediate, arbitrate, or litigate.

Step 1. Organize your contract files. To audit payments and terms, contracts must be readily accessible and located in a central place with easy access to those responsible for auditing. Neatly organized contract files separated by the signed agreement, amendments, and correspondence help the auditor when thumbing through hundreds of contract terms and pages. A separate file for each contract is necessary and should be kept locked and in a safe place. Contracts are assets and can pose problems for the providers if they are lost.

Step 2. Identify key indicators to monitor. Practices should monitor both financial and operational indicators. It is important to make a list of the key indicators and monitor the same ones for all payers. This creates consistency and standardization in the review process.

One example is for the practice manager to use the power of the practice management system to compare the EOB allowable on a large number of paid claims against the expected contract allowable. If the sum of the EOB allowable for all the claims is far from the expected contractual reimbursement, this problem requires further investigation.

It may not be feasible to audit all the codes paid by each payer, but a reasonable conclusion might be drawn from a sample of codes. For example, in many primary care practices, a large proportion of total charges may be aggregated in only 20 CPT codes. These are the codes that should be audited for proper payment.

Most practices receive electronic remittances from payers. Having the computer automatically compare the remittance to the expected allowable is a great way to audit payments.

Other operational indicators include the effective date of the current contract, renewal dates (at least 90 days from notice), termination dates, price increase dates, write offs for noncovered services, timely filing, timely payment, and denials. (Denials include those caused by both the provider and payer with specific denial types. It is critical to have a process in place to track all payer denials until they are resolved.)

Step 3. Track and document discrepancies. This step is critical if you want to justify through data that a trend or problem exists. It is important to identify the clause in the contract that does or does not gain you reimbursement. This will serve to inform the contracting department that wording may need to be revised on the renewal. Reports that summarize auditing problems by category help to communicate not only with the payer, but also with the senior leaders of the practice.

Auditing should be viewed as a program, with monthly and/or quarterly reports listing the payer, audit category, dollars recovered, dollars denied, and dollars pending for recovery. Auditing not only improves the practice's bottom line, but also serves to inform contracting of the changes necessary to prevent the likelihood of further occurrences.

When there is a dispute, it is critical to locate that section in the contract that allows the payer to not pay, and to understand it.

26

Identifying this part of the contract helps the practice better address the issue during the next round of negotiations.

Another strength of payer auditing is that it serves to inform contracting of the issues facing back-end business claims so that specifics can be addressed during contract renegotiations. Real experiences allow the contracting team to ask for things that they might not have known to be problematic in the past.

Step 4. Prepare to mediate, arbitrate, or litigate. Although these methods are never preferred, sometimes they are necessary to reach a resolution. They should be applied judiciously; having a good working relationship with the payer is always desirable. Be sure that all efforts to reach a resolution have been exhausted. Additionally, check the wording in the contract to ensure that you have the right to either arbitration or litigation. Both approaches can be time consuming and costly, so it is important to weigh the costs and benefits of taking such action. When all else fails, a practice may consider terminating the contract.

Developing a Financial Policy for Patient Payments

The practice should develop a financial policy that explains to staff and patients the practice's expectations regarding payments. At a minimum, this policy should include the following:

- Require that patients make their copayments at the time of service;
- Clearly state what the practice will do if the patient does not pay, for example:
  - Will the patient be rescheduled?
  - Will a partial payment be accepted?
  - Who will be notified in the office?
- Require payment of past-due balances within 30 days, including:
  - Spell out consequences if patients fail to pay past balances;

- o Let patients know if the practice will continue to schedule appointments for them; and
- o Provide examples of an acceptable partial payment;
- Provide the circumstances (if any) under which the practice will agree to an extended payment plan with the patient and the policy regarding such plans;
- Describe the terms for discounts for uninsured patients who make payments at the time of service, including:
  - o Does this discount depend on the patient being under a certain income level?
  - o Over what period will payments be extended?
  - o Does the discount only apply if the paid at the time of service?
  - o At what point during the patient encounter will the practice inform patients of its financial policy?
- Handle precertification and patient-due portions; and
- Identify noncovered services and how payments are handled for those services.

Charity Care

Closely related to the financial policy is the practice's charity care policy. Some insured patients may lack the financial resources for copayments, deductibles, or coinsurance. Other patients may be simply unwilling or unable to pay because they may have other financial priorities. The charity care policy needs to differentiate between those situations. Key decisions in developing the charity care policy include:

- The income level and related demographic or financial considerations that define the charity care patient;
- Under what circumstances the practice will see charity care patients; and
- What portion (if any) the practice expects charity care patients to pay.

Developing a charity care policy helps the collection process by first defining the charity care patient. Without criteria, collection becomes a game in which the patients try to convince staff they can't

28

pay. Unfortunately, some who merely have other priorities can often state their case quite persuasively, while others who are truly needy are embarrassed or just give up trying to communicate with the practice.

When a practice fails to define charity care patients at the time of service, substantial time and effort can be expended trying to collect those bills. Identifying charity care patients early lets the practice concentrate its collection efforts on patients who should be able to pay, thus eliminating or substantially reducing its costs trying to collect from patients who are unable to pay their bills.

In connection with identifying charity care patients, the practice may help identify other resources to assist with those patients' medical bills. For example, some may be eligible for Medicaid or other medical assistance programs.

When Insurance Doesn't Cover Claims

As part of the financial policy, the practice should establish policies for identifying noncoverage situations that would apply to their practice. Commercial insurers and government payers do not reimburse providers for all services, such as cosmetic or bariatric procedures provided to their patients. A payer may also limit the frequency with which it will pay for certain procedures, such as Pap smears. Payers may also deny payment for certain services, claiming that they were not medically necessary or were not approved in advance.

Medicare requires the provider to give prior notice to a Medicare patient for noncovered services in order to for the provider to bill the patient for these services. The patient must generally sign the notice form. Medicare has strict rules regarding the content and delivery of the notice called *Advance Beneficiary Notice of Noncoverage (ABN)*, Form CMS-R-131. In most situations, the practice must have genuine doubt that Medicare will not cover the service, and the ABN must identify the reason for noncoverage and estimated cost to the patient.

Other payers may prohibit the provider from collecting from the patient for noncovered services if the provider did not provide notice or follow a particular protocol in arranging for and providing the services. Those situations should be clearly spelled out in the contract or the payer's provider manual.

Patients may act surprised that the services were not covered and refuse to pay the bill, blaming the practice for providing unnecessary services or not properly informing them that services were not covered. Understanding the insurance coverage and handling the financial arrangements and paperwork in advance of performing the services improves both collections and relationships with patients and payers.

Internal and External Collections

Even with a financial policy and skilled front desk team, the practice will inevitably have patient accounts that require extra collection efforts. For most practices, a combination of internal and external debt collection produces the best results. Although an outside collection agency will charge a percentage of what it collects, the practice also consumes internal resources attempting to collect the debts. At some point, the salaries and other practice expenses required to collect exceed the amount collected, so the practice needs to assess its internal collection results and costs vs. those of an agency.

The internal process usually consists of sending monthly statements at 30, 60, and 90 days, followed by a phone call and a collection letter. The practice should track staff costs for these collection efforts to determine the point at which it makes sense to abandon internal collection efforts and turn the account over to an outside agency.

Accounts Receivable Overview

The revenue cycle has the largest effect on a practice's profitability. MGMA Cost Survey data have consistently shown that the more profitable practices are usually those with higher total revenue per full-time equivalent (FTE) physician. The key indicators discussed in this section are useful analytical tools for evaluating revenue cycle performance.

Many are ratios that can be compared with the practice's past performance or industry benchmarks such as the MGMA Cost Survey. Such comparisons are useful in spotting areas in which the practice can improve its financial performance. For example, a low net collection ratio indicates the potential for more profitability by improving collections.

The three main indicators discussed in this section (days in A/R, A/R aging, and net collection ratio) are often referred to as the three leading indicators of billing and collections.

A practice should never focus on improving only one of these indicators when trying to make the revenue cycle more efficient. For example, if a practice rewards employees only for reducing days in A/R, it might discover that success does not translate to increased collections. The employees may have written off amounts that they should have been trying to collect in order to reduce the A/R more expeditiously. Use a holistic approach when formulating policies so that all indicators are taken into account.

Days in Accounts Receivable

Days in A/R is an important benchmark. Also known as *days outstanding collections*, it shows the practice's ability to manage this important asset and turn it into cash. It calculates the average number of days from the date of service to the collection of cash. Here is the typical formula for calculating this benchmark:

Total Accounts Receivable / (Gross Charges/Days in Period)

Because the gross charges amount can vary significantly, depending on the physicians' fee schedule, the industry standard is to view the average daily charge over a year (365 days). This allows easier comparison to external benchmarks, such as those provided in MGMA Cost Surveys.

Days in A/R gives the number of days of charges in the practice's A/R balance, thus indicating how quickly the practice collects its fees. Because the normal accounting cycle lasts one year, the year is most often used in computing available industry benchmarks, including the results of the MGMA Cost Survey. Thus, the average daily charge would be based on the annual gross charges, using the following formula:

Average Daily Charge = Annual Gross Charges / 365

Consider computing the average daily charge for periods other than one year for internal purposes. The average daily charge can be computed for periods of time other than one year by dividing the gross charges for that period by the number of days in that period. When benchmarking to outside data, use the time period used in determining that data.

The practice may find that for purposes of comparing internal data, computations using shorter time periods may be more meaningful. For example, when computing the average daily charge based on annual charges, a practice that has seasonal activity would show an unusually low number of days in A/R for periods of low activity and unusually high number of days in A/R for periods of high activity. This is because the A/R balance (the numerator) fluctuates depending on the level of recent activity, while the average daily gross charge (the denominator) will reflect the annual average. Using a shorter time period (such as the most recent 60 days) to compute the average daily charge provides more current and realistic data.

Another potential pitfall in computing days in A/R happens when a practice computes its average daily gross charges at a single point in time, then continues to use the same denominator to measure days in A/R for successive periods. Doing so could give unrealistic values should practice charge levels change.

For example, assume a practice uses the prior year's daily average charge to compute days in A/R. If the practice experiences a 20 percent increase in its gross charges, then its A/R would be expected to also increase by about 20 percent. If the practice is still measuring its average daily gross charge based on last year's data, then (absent any other changes in its collections or fee schedule) its computed days in

A/R would also increase 20 percent, which would be neither realistic nor provide useful data to the practice.

A high number of days in A/R could indicate:

- Failure to perform timely and effective follow-up on past-due balances;
- Failure to work denials;
- A long charge lag;
- Clean claim problems;
- Failure to collect copayments;
- Failure to turn past-due balances to an outside collection agency on a timely basis;
- Credentialing or contracting issues, such as a new physician; and
- Payers causing delays.

Accounts Receivable Aging

A/R aging is an indicator that gives the percentage of the A/R in the different aging categories as compared to the total A/R. Aging categories normally included in such an analysis are:

- Current–30 days;
- 31–60 days;
- 61–90 days;
- 91–120 days;
- More than 120 days, and;
- Total A/R.

The most frequent comparisons center on the percentage of the A/R that is over 90 or 120 days. Unusually high percentages in those categories indicate that a practice has problems collecting or resolving its charges on a timely basis. Potential reasons for this problem include the collection staff members not working the past-due accounts on a timely basis or not working them effectively and accounts not being turned over to an outside collection agency on a timely basis.

Practice administrators might also want to compare the percentages in their 31–60 and 61–90 days categories. Unusually high percentages in those categories could indicate that:

- Charges are not being entered on a timely basis (see discussion in the "Days Lag to Post Charges" section later in this chapter);
- The practice is not collecting copayments at the time of service;
- The practice may have a large percentage of claims rejected; or
- The practice is experiencing a seasonal lag in collecting due to deductibles.

Large percentages in any of the noncurrent balances might indicate credentialing or contracting problems and economic or demographic issues. Computing percentages by payer can be useful in locating problems with a particular payer or credentialing issues. Aging percentages can vary by specialty.

A computerized practice management system allows the practice to easily produce reports of A/R in these categories and also by payer source, patient, physician, specialty, department, and other classifications. Tracking this data over time — comparing A/R month to month or between the current month and the previous year — provides a useful picture of the practice's collections performance. These snapshots can help the administrator to understand and anticipate cash flow into the practice and spot any potential causes of uncollected debt.

Useful Accounts Receivable Formulas

Net (or Adjusted) Collection Ratio

Your practice's A/R data is only as useful as the methods you use to extract useful information from it. An oft-used formula is:

Net Collection Ratio = Net Collections/(Gross Charges – Contractual Write Offs – Charity Care)

This ratio gives the amount actually collected as a percentage of what was theoretically collectible. The denominator subtracts contractual adjustments and charity care, but not bad debts and other write offs, from gross collections in determining the amount theoretically collectible. This ratio is an important indicator in assessing billing and collection performance.

Gross Collection Ratio

The gross collection ratio is computed as follows:

> **Gross Collection Ratio = Net Collections/Gross Charges**

This indicator computes net collections as a percentage of gross charges. It can be useful in predicting cash receipts and in assessing the reasonableness of the practice's fee schedule. It may also be helpful in payer contract negotiations and assessing contract profitability. Because gross charges (the denominator) depend on the practice's fee schedule, *this ratio is not usually meaningful in assessing billing office performance.* Fee schedules can vary significantly among practices and among the various specialties. A better measure of billing office performance is the net collections ratio discussed above.

When combined with other indicators, the gross collection ratio can sometimes be useful as a catalyst for determining revenue cycle problems. For example, consider a practice that has A/R aging, days in A/R, and an adjusted collection ratio that have remained relatively unchanged over the past year, but the gross collection ratio is down.

This might indicate that:

- Payer contractual reimbursement is down;
- Business office staff are writing off workable denials and/ or patient responsibility as contractual allowances in error; or
- Payers are underpaying, and business office staff is not catching this.

Comparisons of Gross Charges

Practices often track gross charges as a measure of whether their activity levels are increasing or decreasing. This can be useful for internal purposes, provided the practice has not had a change in its fee schedule.

Comparisons of gross charges amounts (including amounts per FTE physician) against external data are generally not meaningful. This amount depends on the fee schedule, which is up to the practice's discretion. The disparity of gross collection ratio amounts among practices and specialties is evidence that fee schedules vary. Comparisons of gross charges by physicians in the practice may not be meaningful if the practice bills a mix of global fees and professional component fees.

Alternative methods of tracking production include the number of procedures, number of patient encounters, number of cases, or number of RVUs. Measuring physician productivity using work RVUs omits factors related to other practice costs, leaving a measurement of physician effort only.

Net Collections

To determine net collections, use the following equation:

> **Net Collections = Gross Collections – (Refunds + Return Checks)**

Net collections are an important revenue cycle indicator. As the amounts actually received by the practice, they are much more real than gross charges. As discussed earlier, revenue tends to drive practice profitability. Thus, practices often track this number. Decreases in net collections are cause for concern.

When computed per FTE physician, this indicator is useful for benchmarking or comparisons with external data. Similar metrics include:

> **Net Fee-for-service Revenue per FTE Physician = Net Fee-for-service Revenue/Number of FTE Physicians**

For cash-based practices, net FFS revenue should equal net collections. Because accrual basis practices recognize revenue when it is earned rather than when it is received, this number will vary somewhat for those practices.

Total Medical Revenue per FTE Physician

To find your total medical revenue per FTE physician, use this equation:

> **Total Medical Revenue per FTE Physician =**
> **Total Medical Revenue ÷ Number of FTE Physicians**

Total medical revenue includes all medical revenue, including net collections (cash) or net fee-for-service revenue (accrual), as well as capitation revenue, sales of pharmaceuticals and medical supplies, revenue from hospital contracts, fees for expert witness testimony, medical goods and services, and so forth.

Accounts Receivable Balance

Practices usually track the balance of their A/R. Some practices track that number as a gross amount, while others (usually accrual basis practices) track the net amount. This provides useful information to the practice regarding up or down trends in the amount. Tracking the net A/R amount provides information regarding estimated future collections.

One knee-jerk reaction to an increase in the practice's A/R balance is to assume that the billing staff is slacking off in its efforts. Although poor performance on the part of the billing office *can* cause an increase in the A/R balance, other factors (some good) can increase that balance. For example, an increase in volume will generally create an increase in both the gross and net A/R balance.

Changes in the practice's fee schedule will affect the gross value of A/R. Because of the discretionary nature of the practice's fee schedule and the variances in those amounts among practices, comparisons of gross A/R balances with external data are not generally meaningful.

Claim Denial Rate

By reducing denials, a practice collects its revenue on the first submission of a claim and avoids the added expense of working the denied claim. Practices are encouraged to track their denial rates and benchmark their success. If a practice's days in A/R are high in relation to external benchmarks, this might be caused by a high claims denial rate.

Days Lag to Post Charges

The longer a practice takes to submit its charges, the higher its A/R balance and the longer the practice waits to receive payment. A long lag in posting charges has a negative effect on the practice's financial indicators. The *charge lag* is the number of days between the date of service and the date the charge was entered in the system. The medical group's practice management system or billing company (if the billing process is outsourced) should be able to compute that amount.

For some practices that depend on hospital registration data, it may not be feasible to wait to submit the charge until receiving the final updates to hospital registration data.

Practices will often experience seasonal trends in practice volume and collections (consistent changes in charge volume and the related net collections) during certain times of the year. Being knowledgeable regarding its seasonal trends enables a practice to better predict its cash flows, prepare a budget, and manage its operations. A practice that does not understand its seasonal variances may become unnecessarily alarmed when charges dip during the holiday season or when collections dip during February, when payers withhold patient deductibles from their remittances.

Why a Good Cutoff Is Important

The practice should ensure that substantially all charges, payments, and adjustments for a particular month are included in that month's activity. Failure to include all of that information can create bad data and misleading indicators, thus impairing the practice's decision-making process.

Some practices are so disciplined about closing the month out immediately that they close out on the last day of the month no matter what. If the practice has a five day lag in posting its charges, then its A/R will be understated by the amount of those charges, and its days in A/R will be understated by five days. When comparing its indicators against external benchmarks, the practice may fail to notice the potential for improvement in its billing and collection processes.

The practice that fails to get a good cutoff lacks decent data with which to compare current month activity with that of the same month during earlier periods. Closing out on the same day each month does not create consistency because internal issues in the billing department, such as staff shortages, staff member illnesses, and technology problems, can create delays in entering data for a particular month. Closing the month without all the data distorts the activity for that month. Knowledge of seasonal variances is useful to practice personnel in anticipating cash flow and evaluating performance.

The Impact of Credit Balances

With the complexity of having to collect from payers, patients, and sometimes secondary payers, the practice inevitably receives overpayments on some of its accounts. Those overpayments result in *credit balances*. Sometimes a practice can get behind in resolving its credit balances, and the aggregate amount can swell to a rather significant number. In some cases, the overpayments are difficult to resolve because payers may disagree with or not respond to the practice's efforts to resolve the problem.

The practice needs to ensure that its staff (or billing company) resolves credit balances and refunds the proper payer within a reasonable period (this may be defined in the practice's contract with the payer). In many cases, failure to do this creates compliance problems.

A large number of unresolved credit balances can create misleading A/R indicators. This is because practices often compute their A/R net of credit balances. If those credit balances are large and old, they decrease not only the total balance of the A/R (and the related days in A/R), they also decrease the aging percentage of the old balances. Thus, the metrics mislead the practice as to the true potential for improved financial performance from revenue cycle initiatives.

Drilling Down to Identify and Address Specific Problems

A practice can benefit from analyzing its revenue cycle indicators on a disaggregated basis, for example, by location, department, physician, payer, or specialty.

Doing so can highlight problems that are not evident when looking at the data for the practice as a whole. For example, by breaking down A/R aging by payer, the practice can locate the payers from whom the practice is having difficulty collecting on a timely basis.

An unusually high percentage of patient balances at a particular location could indicate a failure to collect copayments and past due balances at the front desk. Breaking down denials by location or specialty can help locate the source of a denial problem. For example, one specialty may be experiencing a large number of diagnosis related denials; a particular location may be receiving an unusually large number of denials related to precertification or bad insurance information.

Accounts Receivable Measurement and Management Systems

A medical practice's most important financial asset is its A/R. A/R represents amounts that have been billed to (but not yet paid by) patients and third-party payers such as insurance companies. A/R can also include amounts billed but not yet paid by other revenue sources, such as clinical trial sponsors, medical directorships, and so forth.

Accurately tracking and measuring these future funds allows a manager to understand how well the practice collects this money, both in the aggregate and from each payment source. Tracking A/R also shows how various payment sources perform in relation to each other and to industry benchmarks. This tracking is more than an academic exercise because A/R represents money that is not yet collected and assets that cannot be used, except perhaps as collateral for loans. In most cases, A/R does not earn interest for the medical practice, which means that inflation and overhead costs erode the value of this asset each day that it remains uncollected.

Poor management of A/R results in delayed collections. The longer the delay, the higher the likelihood the accounts will become uncollectible claims that must be written off. Ultimately, poor management of A/R causes a shortage of incoming cash that the practice relies on to pay staff and providers, service debt, and attend to its other financial obligations. Inaccurate tracking of A/R reduces the practice's ability to anticipate its future cash flow and spot ways to improve its coding, billing, and collections processes. Therefore, it is critical that new charges for services rendered are posted in a timely manner, billing is sent to payers and patients expeditiously, and revenues are reported accurately. Protocols must be created and enforced to conduct credit checks and investigations, when appropriate, and ensure accurate and clear billing and collection policies.

Benchmarking

Benchmarking helps managers monitor and analyze the practice's financial and operational performance. Benchmarking data can be extracted from a variety of sources, but it most frequently comes from the practice's computerized practice management system. By measuring this data across time — internally among different people and processes, as well as against industry benchmark — a practice manager can develop a clear road map for process improvement.[13]

Several internal and external benchmarks are commonly tracked and analyzed for A/R. These benchmarks include total days in A/R and days receivables outstanding, both of which were discussed previously in this chapter. Monitoring the practice's performance in days in A/R and the percent of A/R in various categories against benchmarks can also help administrators decide when to write off A/R as uncollectible.[14]

Net vs. Gross Revenue

Revenue, which is the inflow of assets (usually cash or receivables) in return for services rendered, increases the practice's net assets and the practice owners' equity. However, it is important to distinguish between net and gross revenue. In a medical practice, gross revenue is the amount expected to be received for services delivered to patients as well as from items, supplies, and other sources including the technical component of radiology procedures, margins from outpatient drugs, and other services. Subtracted from gross revenue are payers' contractual allowances, sliding fee discounts, and other adjustments.

Regulatory Agency and Contract Guidelines and Mandates

Several federal agencies regulate the financial aspects of medical practice reimbursement from public insurance programs such as Medicare and Medicaid. Private insurers also develop reimbursement guidelines that may vary from those of the public programs. In addition, several nonpublic agencies promulgate voluntary quality standards and accreditation requirements that the healthcare industry recognizes. These standards may influence private payers' and, increasingly, consumers' decisions to select a hospital or medical practice.

Centers for Medicare & Medicaid Services

CMS, a federal agency within the U.S. Department of Health and Human Services, administers the Medicare and Medicaid programs that provide health insurance coverage to approximately 135 million Americans.[15] Formerly known as the Health Care Financing Administration, the role of CMS in the regulatory oversight of physicians and other providers is significant because many physicians and hospitals accept Medicare beneficiaries and rely on those medical revenues.

Because of the size of its insured population, the agency's rules and payment policies often set the tone for the policies of private insurance companies. Efforts by CMS to protect the fiscal integrity of its programs and ensure appropriate and predictable payments and high-quality care have led to many regulations of which the practice administrator must be aware. Violating these rules can result in fines, civil or criminal actions, and temporary or permanent expulsion from participating in Medicare and Medicaid programs, as well as from the State Children's Health Insurance Program, which CMS also administers. The agency is also responsible for overseeing the Health Insurance Portability and Accountability Act (HIPAA) administrative simplification transaction and code sets, health identifiers, and security standards.

Insurance

Private insurance companies may set payment policies within the broader outlines of state and federal regulations. The medical practice manager must ensure that the practice follows the reimbursement, coding, and collection policies of its many private insurance payers. Failure to abide by a private insurer's rules can result in denied claims, but may also bring other penalties, such as exclusion from that insurer's network or cancellation of its contracts with the provider. Private insurance companies may also seek civil action against providers who violate their billing and coding guideline rules. In cases where a payer suspects fraud, the payer may have grounds to seek civil or criminal prosecution by public authorities.

State Regulations

States create guidelines for healthcare quality and business practices through laws and regulations. These rules may affect the corporate structure of a medical practice as well as how it operates and what revenue opportunities it may explore. A state also may regulate the business practices of health insurance companies doing business in the state. In addition, states set scope of practice laws that determine what services nonphysician providers may provide to patients of a medical practice.

43

Healthcare Effectiveness Data and Information Set

The National Committee for Quality Assurance (NCQA) developed HEDIS. HEDIS is a tool that consists of a set of performance measures for managed care organizations. These measures, such as immunization and mammography screening rates, can show how well health plans perform in the areas of quality of care and access to care. HEDIS also measures member satisfaction with the health plan and its doctors. Health plans collect these data in a standardized manner and must have their HEDIS results verified by independent auditors. Although it is not mandated by law, the use of HEDIS has become a more widely accepted tool for health insurance purchasers to gauge the quality of care and service a health plan provides. More than half the nation's HMOs currently participate in order to gain an NCQA seal of approval, and close to 90 percent of all health plans measure performance using HEDIS.[16]

National Committee for Quality Assurance

NCQA is a private, not-for-profit organization that establishes standards of quality in management care plans and reports these outcomes to the public. To gain NCQA accreditation, a health plan must self-monitor its performance on the HEDIS measures that NCQA develops and take steps to improve performance. As a nongovernmental agency, the NCQA does not have legal power to discipline noncompliant organizations, but rather it can grant or withhold its accreditation. NCQA makes its assessments available on the web (at www.healthchoices.org and www.ncqa.org) for employers and the public to make healthcare purchasing decisions. The organization plans to issue ratings of medical groups and individual physicians.

The Joint Commission

The Joint Commission (formerly the Joint Commission on Accreditation of Healthcare Organizations or JCAHO) is a not-for-profit organization that evaluates and accredits more than 20,500 healthcare organizations and programs in the United States.[17] Its goal is to improve the quality and safety of care provided by healthcare organizations. The

Joint Commission's accreditation process evaluates an organization's compliance with standards and other accreditation requirements. Its voluntary evaluation and accreditation services are provided to hospitals, long and short-term care facilities, home healthcare agencies, laboratories, group practices, ambulatory surgery centers, and organizations that deliver disease management and chronic care services. The accreditation process requires inspections at least every three years.

Coding Systems, Guidelines, and Resources

Payers, including the Medicare program, apply various payment guidelines to reimburse physicians for services they render to patients. These guidelines rely on published numerical codes that a provider enters on an electronic or paper encounter form to indicate the medical diagnosis and the resulting services, procedures, or supplies that are rendered. Practices must establish standards for proper documentation and coding to ensure that billing is accurate and complete. Improper coding and documentation can cause overpayments, underpayments, and denials of claims.

The authors of *The Physician Billing Process: Navigating Potholes on the Road to Getting Paid, 3rd edition*[18] suggest making coding and billing resources available to providers, managers, and staff to ensure that coding standards are understood and followed. Such resources would include:

- The current CPT codebook (updated each January);
- ICD-10-CM, and additional manuals for certain specialties (updated each October);
- The current HCPCS manual (updated each January);
- The National Correct Coding Initiative (NCCI) coding edits;,
- National and local coverage determinations;
- Information regarding MIPS/MACRA quality reporting;
- A medical dictionary;
- Medicare and/or Medicaid regional carrier updates and any specialty billing guides (kept electronically or on paper in a binder);

- Insurance newsletters;
- Medical specialty publications; and
- Online access to the *Federal Register* (www.thomas.loc. gov), CMS (www.cms.gov), the state Medicaid program website, and insurance company websites.[18]

CPT and ICD-10-CM

Most payers, including CMS, which administers the Medicare program, process claims for medical services using CPT codes. The American Medical Association (AMA) maintains this coding structure, which it developed and copyrighted, and produces both a professional and standard version of the codebook each year along with peripheral materials. Using the AMA CPT codebooks, five digit codes can be assigned to medical services and procedures as a way to standardize claims processing and data analysis. CPT codes may have modifiers attached so the provider can provide more detail when needed. Although CPT codes identify the medical services provided, they do not name payment amounts. Payers choose which codes they will reimburse, specify when those codes and modifiers are reimbursable, and set payment amounts for codes.

The HCPCS is a standardized method used to report professional services, procedures, and supplies. HCPCS codes are typically paid on a flat rate and not assigned RVUs (relative measurements of work effort). HCPCS codes are used to identify services not fully described in the CPT system, such as ambulance transportation, injections, durable medical equipment, and supplies. They are also used for new procedures not yet assigned CPT codes. Some HCPCS codes, also known as *Level III HCPCS codes* or *local codes*, may be used in certain states or regions at the discretion of the regional Medicare carrier or the state's Medicaid program.

Payers also require physicians and other providers to supply one or more diagnosis codes to justify the procedures for which they are claiming reimbursement. The diagnosis codes, which are alphanumeric, are listed in the ICD-10-CM. The National Center for Health Statistics and CMS oversee modifications of ICD-10-CM, which are based on an internationally agreed on methodology to track diseases and injuries.

ICD-10-CM codes are three to seven digits long, depending on the level of specificity. These codes identify diagnoses, symptoms, conditions, or other reasons for an encounter or visit. There are ICD-10-CM codes that also represent causes of injury as well as codes that represent for general health status exams.

Evaluation and Management Levels of Service

Evaluation and management (E&M) codes are listed in the AMA CPT codebooks and tend to represent the cognitive services that physicians perform. The CPT E&M codes apply to:

- Office visits;
- Hospital visits;
- Consultations;
- Emergency services;
- Critical care; and
- Other services, such as home services, case management, and telemedicine.

Each of these areas has as many as five levels of care, from simple to complex. When these areas are fully documented, they reflect the physicians' work and help determine reimbursement amounts.

CMS has created documentation guidelines to help physicians understand how to apply codes for E&M services. These guidelines are available on the CMS website. Six of the seven components below are used in defining the level of E&M service. The first three (history, exam, medical decision making) are considered the key components for E&M selection. The next three (counseling, coordination of care, nature of the presenting problem) are contributing factors in a majority of encounters. The use of time to determine the level of E&M has its own specific documentation requirements.

The seven components to determine the proper level of coding:

1. History;
2. Examination;

3. Medical decision making;

4. Counseling;

5. Coordination of care;

6. Nature of presenting problem; and

7. Time.

The degree to which these components are satisfied helps determine, for example, whether an office visit is coded as a simple encounter (i.e., a CPT coded 99211 visit) or a more complex (and likely a more highly reimbursed) encounter, such as a 99215.

Charge Capturing, Billing, and Collection Systems

The process of capturing (recording) the charge for the service rendered to the patient and then billing and collecting for it might seem straight forward, but it is error prone in many practices. Some practices may still rely on paper forms to capture charges in both the hospital and office settings where the providers encounter patients. This capture process may be based on dictated reports, paper forms, handwritten notes, or data entered into computer software programs. Unfortunately, errors in developing the fee schedule, auditing the capture of charges, or ensuring that efficient billing and collection processes are followed may cause charge entries to be incomplete or sometimes not made at all. Thus, the practice cannot receive the full reimbursement for the services its physicians and other providers have rendered.[19]

Patient Encounter Records

These practices find that a well-designed encounter form, whether it is in paper or electronic form, is an efficient way to help the physician quickly and accurately capture the appropriate procedure and diagnosis codes. Physicians usually complete this form during or immediately after an encounter with a patient. The encounter form is an internal document that should be customized for the practice and include the current procedure and diagnosis codes used most frequently by the physicians.[20] A logical layout of information to check off on the form lets the physician quickly select CPT and ICD-10 codes, document the level of service, and make brief notes. The form can also list fees for various services. The form can be used as a receipt for the patient, to track physician laboratory orders, and to communicate follow-up appointment recommendations. Most importantly, the form becomes a document of the encounter that can be used to initiate the billing process. Along with the form, more complete documentation is placed into the patient's chart, either electronically or in writing.

Month End Closing

The process of ending a financial reporting period is called *closing the books*. This means that billing staff does not enter any new information for the period, unless it is a correction or restatement of previously gathered data. Charges dated in the current period that were not entered before the month end closing would be included with those of the period in which they were subsequently entered. (Although it is important to enter charges in the correct period, it is more important that they get billed.) Discounts, payments, or other adjustments to accounts outstanding received after the applicable month's ledger is closed should be entered in the ledger for the month in which they were actually received.

Electronic Claims Processing

Electronic claims processing is the electronic submission of claims to payers or clearinghouses that reformat the data and retransmit it to the appropriate insurance company or fiscal intermediary. Once a rare option, electronic submission is now a given in most cases.

Effective in 2005, all claims for services to Medicare beneficiaries were required be transmitted to the program in a format that complied with HIPAA electronic transactions standards.[21] Following the lead of the Medicare program, most private insurance companies also require medical practices to submit claims electronically. Many medical practices dealt with this challenge by upgrading their internal billing systems to submit HIPAA-compliant electronic claims directly to Medicare and payers. Practices that had already invested in a practice management system that could produce electronic claims in compliance with the HIPAA-standard electronic transactions standards use clearinghouses to translate their claims into the HIPAA-standard formats.

Practices that want to continue using paper-based billing are faced with the more expensive and time-consuming process of sending paper claims to a billing service where they are converted into an electronic format. The billing service sends the converted claims to a clearinghouse that translates them to the HIPAA-standard format and then, finally, the claims are sent to payers. Today most claims are sent electronically. The fact that Medicare and other payers require electronic claims processing is not the only reason to use this technology. Other benefits are that electronic processing lets the practice:

- Edit (and correct) claims before submitting them to payers;
- Generate productivity reports;
- Reduce rebilling; and
- Improve cost effectiveness in billing.

Collection Agency Policy

A collection agency can be an important component of an effective collections program for medical practices. Traditionally, medical groups outsource delinquent accounts to professional collectors after a significant period of time, such as 120 or more days.

Before referring delinquent accounts to an agency for collection, the practice manager should consider whether:

- Agency fees are reasonable compared with internal collection costs;
- The probability of collection is greater using an agency than using internal resources;

- The account is uncollectible, both practically and legally, because many payers set time limits on collections of patient balances; and
- Public relations will suffer. Collections efforts, however polite and courteous, may arouse a patient's anger. An agency may have personnel better equipped to handle collections than the medical practice, but any problems an agency causes will hurt the practice's public image.

When selecting a third party to service accounts, the most important element to consider is the financial integrity of the agency. This is best indicated by a long record of ethical dealings with other clients, particularly medical group practices and other healthcare providers. Additional factors to consider when selecting an agency are:

- Accurate accounting and recording of all funds collected for other medical group clients;
- Prompt remittance of those collections;
- Awareness of public or patient relations;
- Willingness to respond to special requests and provide reports;
- Net recovery rate;
- Understanding of the special nature of medical accounts;
- References, such as the names of other companies, medical institutions, and professional people whom the agency is servicing; and
- Commissions, in that agencies usually accept accounts for collection on a contingency basis; that is, no collection, no charge. Contingent fee commissions range from 25 to 40 percent.

Accounts previously handled by other agencies, those that require legal action, and accounts transferred to out-of-town agencies may put the fee at a higher percentage.

To monitor how a collection agency handles your accounts, routinely review the following reports:

- Collection agency performance — This report shows the collection agency's current and year-to-date collections and the total amount of possible collection balances pending.
- Aged trial balance by collection agency — This report shows the aging of accounts listed for collection by date of listing.
- Unpaid accounts submitted to collection agency — This report reflects all accounts submitted to a collection agency prior to 90 days and showing no subsequent payment. This time frame is arbitrary; it may be valuable to review several such reports with varying time limits.

Collection Letters

Form letters are not as effective for collecting healthcare dollars as they were years ago. Statements, letters, and notices generated by a computer must be constructed to provide a payoff. Careful design is important to ensure best results, both in collection and in public relations. Some useful guidelines to follow are:

- Keep collection letters short and to the point;
- Use letters to follow up on small balance accounts (telephone calls remain more productive when dealing with insurance companies that owe for large account balances); and
- Keep collection notices and statements simple. Include all information regarding the account — date of service, balance, and account number — on the notice and statements. Also include a return envelope. If the group accepts credit cards, be sure to clearly state this payment option.

Telephone Collection

If sending three or four notices by mail to a patient with a delinquent account is not effective, then conduct a follow-up telephone call. The practice can effectively do this follow-up; however, the staff members assigned to this task should be experienced and well trained. An overly aggressive approach will not only produce negative public relations, if performed by a debt collection agency on behalf of the practice, it could also violate the Fair Debt Collection Practices Act, which is enforced both administratively and judicially. The Federal Trade Commission can treat a violation of the act as an unfair and deceptive practice under the law. Violators are subject to civil penalties in federal and state courts.

If the collection effort is targeted at a payer who may have several outstanding delinquencies, then staff members making these calls should receive reports of aged trial balances arranged by the guarantor or responsible party. These reports can help in the telephone follow-up effort because all the payer's delinquent accounts can be referenced in the same call.

Collection Follow-Up

The account collection process for payment of patient balances involves sending multiple statements to patients after both the primary and any secondary insurance companies have paid their portions of the bill. Practices often choose to send a certain number of statements, such as three, and if the account still remains unpaid, they follow up by taking additional actions such as making telephone calls and/or sending collection letters. Practices should develop these steps as part of a comprehensive collection follow-up process to ensure that fair and effective collection steps are attempted before turning the account over to a collection agency. To ensure that internal collection efforts are consistent with the practice's overall style and patient satisfaction goals, the practice administrator may wish to:

- Create protocols and a code of ethics for collections;
- Identify and thoroughly train staff members who will be assigned to make patient collection calls;
- Consistently follow timelines for sending collection letters and turning over an account to a collection agency;
- Establish payment plan options;

- Advise and seek all patients' signed consent to the practice's written collections policy, preferably when patients make their first visits to the practice;
- Attempt to collect past due amounts when patients visit the office;
- Remind patients of past due amounts when they call to schedule appointments;
- Develop and use a charity care policy for patients experiencing hardship; and
- Follow standard industry practices of declaring A/R uncollectible before outsourcing it to a collection agency but continue monitoring those collections efforts.

Disputes

The practice should carefully develop a written protocol for handling billing disputes with patients. This protocol should designate a trained and experienced member of the staff to handle these situations.

Bankruptcy Claims

Practices should be aware of applicable federal and state laws concerning whether and how the practice may continue to pursue unpaid amounts after a patient files for personal bankruptcy protection. Practices normally write off these amounts as uncollectible.

Settlements

After internal and external collections and negotiations for payments fail, some medical practices choose to pursue unpaid accounts, especially ones with large balances. In many states, the amounts owed may fall within the limits of small claims courts; typically, a magistrate hears these cases and there is no jury. If the practice prevails in court, the practice is responsible for collecting the judgment. Once payment is received or the practice is satisfied that it has collected all that is possible, it must file a creditor's Satisfaction of Judgment, which tells the court that the case is closed. If the practice does not receive payment, it can ask the court to order the debtor to identify his or her assets for possible liquidation. The magistrate can issue a warrant to require the debtor to respond to this inquiry or face imprisonment for failure to respond. However, the debtor cannot be imprisoned for failure to pay the judgment. With a court judgment, it is possible to garnish the patient's wages. This requires his or her employer to pay the county sheriff as much as 25 percent of the individual's paycheck, which the sheriff then forwards to your practice. Physicians should check their state's judicial branch website for more information.

Time Payments (Budgeted Payments)

An important step to ensure timely collection of receivables is to grant credit to self pay patients who have a good credit history and fully accept your payment terms. Many practices provide a range of payment terms. The patient agrees to a particular payment plan and the receivables system reports any deviations from the plan. A patient who agrees to pay in 30 days should be considered delinquent after 60 days. Make sure any automated systems can recognize the various payment terms. For example, a patient may not have paid an account in full at the end of 30 days because the agreement was to pay in three installments over three months. Teach staff to handle patients who wish to make special payment arrangements. When possible, attempt to secure the payment arrangement with the responsible party before the service is provided. A receptionist at the front desk or a cashier at the checkout desk who has access to account information can increase collections and reduce later collection problems. The after-service interview could be a last chance situation. Even if the patient is returning at a future date, this could be the last convenient opportunity to complete records with information not previously collected. Also, it may be the only opportunity to place a bill before the patient and attempt to collect the balance. Tight control and knowledge of charges and payments are crucial to good cash flow.

One means of helping to ensure collections on payment plans spanning multiple months is to set up authorizations to charge the patient's credit card or debit the patient's bank account for these payments. Practices using these arrangements must comply with applicable federal and state laws regarding agreements with the patient, securing the credit card/bank account information, notification, and any other applicable laws. The vendor holding the card information must be PCI DSS (Payment Card Industry Data Security Standards) compliant.

Another tool for improving cash flow in medical groups is to let a financial institution carry patient accounts that need monthly payments. Ideally, practices should avoid contract payments on large balances. Collecting these large amounts a little at a time will tie up cash, require more collection follow-up, and will likely be too costly. Since charging interest has never been a viable alternative for healthcare receivables, alternative methods to handle accounts that would require long term monthly payments are to accept credit card payments or bank financing.

Write Offs

There is a temptation to write off an account instead of referring it to a third-party for collection. This approach has three drawbacks.

1. **Word might get around of the medical group's unwillingness to take all possible steps to collect payment.** A reputation of this nature can lead to more chronic debtor nonpayment, thus increasing collection costs considerably.

2. **This approach is not fair to paying patients.** In the long run, someone must pay for those who do not. An indirect result may be increased charges for all patients. In today's environment, holding down costs must be a prime consideration.

3. **Medicare regulations require that a practice make a reasonable attempt to collect funds due.** Medicare typically defines attempts as reasonable by considering the amount owed vs. the cost to collect. (In other words, a practice isn't required to try to collect if the attempt costs more than the amount to be collected.) If the balance owed is high, and the practice consistently

writes such balances off after sending out a few bills and making some calls, the amount owed may have been greater than the cost to collect. Medicare and other payers may view this consistent practice of writing off accounts as a standard discount percentage and uniformly reduce the allowances to the practice.

Developing Reconciliation Systems for Third-Party Payments

The practice revenue cycle extends from day of service, through billing patients and insurance companies, to the actual collection of the cash. Ideally, all services would be paid in cash on the day of service. In reality, most practices send a charge ticket to a billing office where the charges are electronically billed to the patient or an insurance company. This process creates an A/R on the practice's books to be collected and reconciled. The collection and reconciliation of payments is the focus of this section.

The practice's A/R are frequently the largest asset on the books. The loss of even a few percent of A/R can add up to large amounts over time. The cost of implementation and maintenance of an effective denial management and audit program will usually more than pay for itself in improved collections.

Payment Policies

Although practice payment policies are generally related to self-pay patients, the implementation of these policies and educating staff on these policies are part of the practice's overall reimbursement procedure. Accounting for bad debt, collection company submission and recoveries, uninsured write offs, and payment plans all have to be addressed in the practice's payment policies for accurate accounting and evaluating A/R collection efficiency. Remember that all must take anti-kickback and Stark laws into account to remain compliant.

Contracting

Many practice managers sometimes consider payer contract analysis and negotiation to be a difficult process with a low probability of success. At the same time, payer contracting is a most critical aspect of the practice revenue cycle. Even if a practice is unable to successfully negotiate rates it believes are fair market, numerous other provisions in the contract, if left unclear or ambiguous (i.e., obligations of the provider to adhere to medical management and care processes or bill timely and accurately), could further erode reimbursement and adversely affect much needed practice revenue. Many practices, especially smaller ones, choose to not read contracts because they are lengthy and contain little opportunity for negotiating. Administrators should read contracts completely and then communicate to the various departments, such as nursing, registration, billing, and collections, so key members of the practice understand their respective obligations for meeting the terms of the contract. As much as 20 percent of revenue can be lost through noncompliant activities, from denials to bundling of codes.

Contract Management

While some general themes can be applied to contracting, almost every situation is different to some degree. These differences most frequently relate to the marketplace and the relative strengths and weaknesses of the negotiating parties. Yet there are many details to manage during the contracting process. To create discipline and reinforce consistency, practices can follow a suggested framework, which will improve negotiations and help to effectively manage multiple payer agreements. The five steps in this framework are:

1. Preparation;
2. Negotiation;
3. Implementation;
4. Operations; and
5. Auditing.

When viewed as part of a cycle, each of these five steps builds and improves on the next step. So, once a practice has audited reimbursement, the preparation for the next round of negotiations is made easier because issues are better understood. Data is integral for effective contract negotiations and, if applied correctly, the process takes discipline. In this section, we will discuss Steps 1 and 2.

Step 1: Preparation

Getting organized is essential, and there are many ways to approach that task. Creating a checklist of items to follow through on during the process helps to ensure that all tasks are completed and establishes discipline into what can be a time consuming, overwhelming process. Additionally, knowledgeable practice managers who come prepared to the negotiating table establish credibility with the health plan.

The practice manager's initial action is to evaluate the relative strengths and weaknesses of the practice and the payers in the negotiation arena. Critical questions that the manager should ask include:

- What is the practice's relative level of dominance in its market? Does the practice feature a physician specialty or subspecialty with little or no competition?
- Is the level of patient and/or incoming referral satisfaction so high that an insurance payer is compelled to include the practice in its provider panel?
- Does the practice have special programs, such as disease management, evening hours, weekend clinics, hospitalist coverage, and so forth, which many patients and payers find attractive and unique?
- How important are the practice and the payer to the employers and health insurance brokers in your community? What other practice strengths and weaknesses could affect negotiations?
- What types of products do the health plans sell?

Second, the practice manager should evaluate the payer organization using a parallel set of questions. After evaluating the medical group's and payer's positions in the marketplace, the manager is in a much better position to evaluate the contract terms and prepare for negotiations.

Third, the practice manager should develop a set of guiding principles that inform the contracting team and process. An assessment reflecting the level of risk the practice is willing to accept (both financial and nonfinancial) helps identify "must haves" vs. "wants." If a practice knows that costs are increasing by 5 percent, one guiding principle may be to require a 5 percent weighted increase on all negotiations, either through utilization changes or rate increases. Including key nurses, physicians, and business staff when creating guiding principles serves to communicate negotiating details, and in the event the practice chooses to walk from a contract, key practice staff is involved.

Fourth, the practice manager should obtain financial information on the practice. Before the negotiations begin with the insurance plan, the practice manager should have a thorough understanding of the current profitability and issues associated with each contract. In fact, most of the work should occur before negotiations actually begin with the insurance company. Completing a payer assessment of some type allows different departments to weigh in on the performance of the payer, in areas such as business services, patient registration, clinical care, and referral management. Additionally, a complete review that includes patient volume by product, utilization by type, and product profitability vs. overall profitability is critical to establishing a complete picture of the payer's performance. As a rule of thumb, you cannot negotiate effectively unless you understand your baseline and know what to ask for.

Of course, this information might not be available for a new contract; in this case, the practice may be wise to refuse an evergreen clause (language indicating that the contract renews automatically unless one party gives notice) until the insurance company proves themselves. Practices typically have more leverage with new payers than they realize. Entrants into the marketplace have the added pressure of establishing new networks; they need providers more than they need insurance companies.

Step 2: Negotiating Contract Language

Negotiating rates is only one component of the overall request. Negotiating risky language out of the contract, as well as removing ambiguous and vague language, is critical to ensuring that the contract performs as is understood. One way is to redline the contract with preferred language. Additionally, clarifying ambiguous language beforehand may allow the practice to obtain desired changes without negotiating them. Because many sections of a contract require scrutiny and negotiation, the practice may want to seek legal counsel.

Areas of risk in contracts are:

- **Type of plan and the payers.** Identifying the products included in the contract helps to clarify and document the rates by product. If it is necessary, and to limit any reimbursement confusion later when claims are audited, attach an exhibit to the agreement that lists the product name and rates. Get a copy of each card and plan description. You will want to separate insurance codes and rates for each product to better monitor volume, denials, and so forth. Ensure that indemnity business is not tied to your HMO or PPO rates; it should be reimbursed at 100 percent of billed charges because it is not being directed to your group. It is also important to have strong definitions of who is the payer, plan, participant, and so on. Weak definitions can cause health plans to sell their network to other payers and apply any rates. Silent and vague contract language is too risky; it is better to capture intent and seek clarity and conciseness.

- **Medical necessity.** Make sure the contract specifies who makes clinical decisions; for example, is it the physician or the plan's director? If it is the plan director, ask for language that allows both your medical director and the plan director to meet and discuss when there is a disagreement. In no way should the plan be allowed to deny the claim for medical necessity if you received prior authorization. For Emergency Medical Treatment and Labor Act cases, the medical director decides medical necessity because the physician is accountable to treat and stabilize a patient under federal law.

- **Indemnification.** The words "hold harmless" are a red flag for signer, so beware! Plans like to include this way of making sure physicians hold the plan harmless for their actions. The contract language should be reciprocal, however, so both parties hold each other harmless and indemnify the acts of each other.

- **Claims payment.** It is critical to understand your state and federal laws for claims payment, particularly when the contract defaults to language governed by state law. Because self-funded plans do not have to comply with state laws, you need to specify time frames.

- **Provider manual.** The operational details of the contract are contained in the provider manual. Payers are increasingly scaling back on the contract and adding to the provider manual. Stipulate that the plan makes no material changes to the provider manual without your written agreement, particularly on material items such as rate changes or medical management obligations.

- **Termination and renewal.** Contracts commonly contain clauses that automatically renew the agreement for another year. It is preferable to have one-year agreements with the top five payers (those responsible for 70 percent of payments to the practice), so language and rates can be renegotiated. This approach requires the practice to set up a tickler system to manage the renewal dates. If this is impossible, consider language that allows for a 90 day out no cause.

- **Access to records.** Payers frequently need to review medical records. Although this need is appropriate, sometimes contained in this provision are access rights to financial information not found on the CMS-1500 claim form, such as costs, and so forth. Avoid language such as "all" patient financial records.

- **Appeals and denials.** If this section is not in the contract, review the provider manual. This area is increasingly important to understand. Because of requirements of prompt pay statutes to settle all claims within 30 to 45 days, payers automatically deny claims to meet their obligation under the law, thus forcing practices to use the denial process. Negotiating reasonable time frames for appealing and settling claims is critical to the practice's cash flow. As a negotiating tactic, track the frivolous denial, quantify the dollars, divide the amount by the payer's RVU, and inform the payer of the additional amount it will cost to contract with the practice because of the added costs of reprocessing unnecessary denials.

- **Compensation.** Specifying the payment type in the agreement is critical to being able to later audit payment correctness, so spell out rates for cases, immunizations, and lab work, and, if possible, create a list of claims scenarios for proof-of-claims hierarchy payment and attach it to the agreement. If the practice is paid on an RBRVS, list the conversion factor year, RVU year, and whether or not it has been adjusted for the three geographic practice cost indices (work, practice expense, and malpractice). It is preferable to use current RVUs and negotiate off a conversion rate. Remove "lesser of" language from agreements, unless you understand where the fee schedule is set and how reimbursement will be affected. The argument to the health plan is that if the contract is based on agreed on rates, the payer should not be able to change them later, because this would affect the modeling of profitability of the contract. At the same time, be careful of usual and customary language in commercial contracts. Embedded in the calculation of usual and customary rates are reimbursement rates for workers' compensation, Medicaid, and Medicare. If the agreement states it is the lesser of usual and customary or the contracted rate, exactly what is included in reimbursement may be unclear.

- **Governing law.** Make sure the governing law is in the state in which the physicians practice. Some of the national networks indicate their home state. This is not feasible for arbitration and claims payment and medical management requirements.

Reviewing contract language is a time-consuming, tedious process, but it is one that will produce better outcomes for the practice. Remember, it's not just about negotiating the rate; language that is disastrous to the practice affects the net margin every time.

Before arranging for a meeting with a payer, the practice manager should be sure that he or she understands all these areas, as well as the payer and its performance. The practice administrator should then arrive at the negotiations with a prepared proposal that includes rates and contract language.

Contract Negotiations: Techniques and Tactics

Effectively negotiating contracts is both an art and a science. The most skillful negotiators are not only extremely prepared and savvy, they balance their knowledge of the practice's needs with respect for the payer's position. Negotiating contracts is about building and maintaining relationships. Because at some point after the negotiations have ended, problems need resolving and a positive relationship between the practice and the payer facilitates this process.

The following recommendations are not intended to be all inclusive but are suggestions to start and build a comfort level with what is considered a difficult process by many managers.

- **Be prepared with data.** The side with the most data to support its position doesn't always win, but preparation can be an advantage. As mentioned earlier, bring a checklist of items to help guide the discussions. Some requests may be standard contract items and others may be specific to the practice's past experience — both positive and negative — with the health plan.

- **Meet face to face if you can.** When people meet face to face, something happens that cannot occur in a phone conversation. The practice has a better chance of getting what it wants, establishing a relationship, and putting together a contract in a face-to-face meeting with the payer. Time should be used wisely, however, so come to negotiations prepared to discuss the details of the deal. Also, take good notes and document the intent of the parties, so you have material to review when it comes to committing the concepts to writing.

- **Be aware of your negotiating style and how it is seen by the other party.** Are you too loud and demanding or excessively meek and mild? What can you expect from the other negotiating party — cooperation or combat?

- **Stay focused on your objectives and goals.** Goal setting should occur jointly between the provider and payer. Understanding the other party's interests and issues helps create a better contract. For example, the payer may not be able to give you a rate increase, but it may be able to give you something else that is important, such as added providers or services that were not previously covered. Although the rate per se didn't increase, the overall value and profitability may have increased. Sometimes, changing contract language and provider obligations is more important than anything else.

- **Define the deal breakers.** What is absolutely necessary for the contract to work? What can be conceded? It's important to recognize that negotiations begin once offers have been made. It is not mandatory to negotiate if an offer is favorable. At times it is preferable to let the payer make the first offer; this allows insights into where it believes the market competitive rates lie.

- **Be professional.** Using courtesy, negotiate only on a win–win basis. Show a genuine interest in the payer's position. Do not allow yourself to become emotional in the negotiating process; one way to do this is to negotiate as a team.

- **Be inventive.** It is one of the most useful assets a negotiator can learn, but it requires looking at the entire package being offered.

- **Persevere.** If the practice doesn't get what it wants, keep it on the list and ask for it again and again. People may change, but the practice's issues may not.

Credentialing of Providers with Contract Payers

The practice will need to complete forms for the payer that give information about the group and its providers, such as medical training, board certification, license numbers, hospital affiliations, malpractice history, National Provider Identifier (NPI) numbers), and continuing education. The practice will generally need to submit this information in connection with the initial contract, and periodically thereafter, typically every one to three years. The practice usually needs to provide similar information when applying for or renewing hospital privileges or malpractice insurance.

This process is referred to as *credentialing*. The practice should designate an individual responsible for credentialing. This individual should maintain a set of files on each provider that contains:

- Copies of medical licenses;
- Copies of degrees and board certification;
- Copies of malpractice certificates;
- Documentation regarding continuing education;

- Curricula vitae;
- Copies of letter assigning the NPI;
- Copies of letters notifying acceptance or renewal of participating provider status, such as from Medicare, Medicaid, and commercial payers;
- Copies of credentialing forms completed in the past; and
- Any other pertinent information generally requested by the practice's payers, malpractice carrier, or facilities.

Getting new providers credentialed on a timely basis is important. The practice generally cannot get paid for new providers' services until those forms are completed, processed, and approved.

That is part of the administrative workload involved in adding a new physician to the practice. Credentialing a new physician normally takes from one to five months, depending on the carrier, the time of year, and whether the physician is new to the state.

Credentialing can take longer in the summer and around the holiday season when the credentialing committees do not meet as frequently.

This process may also take longer when the practice is hiring a physician from another state who must generally become licensed in the new practice's state before beginning the credentialing process with payers.

To help streamline the credentialing process, the practice should consider developing a checklist of the information it will need from new providers and giving it to them as early as possible in order to get their hospital affiliations, malpractice coverage, and participating provider status as soon as possible (and thus get paid sooner). The practice should also develop a summary sheet of standard credentialing data for all providers, such as address, license numbers, important dates, and so forth.

The Council for Affordable Healthcare (CAQH) provides an online database that helps streamline the credentialing process. Providers set up an account with CAQH and provide pertinent information and required documentation. So, rather than the practice providing this same information to multiple insurance companies, the insurance companies can obtain this information directly from CAQH. Some insurance companies require that providers use CAQH as a condition for enrollment and participation.

The credentialing process — having to provide the same information to multiple parties on separate forms — is redundant and frequently cited as an example of administrative complexity in the U.S. healthcare system. However, mastering that credentialing process will improve the practice's revenue cycle.

Conclusion

The effective management of the revenue cycle may be the single most important component of a practice administrator's job. Clearly, this process is complex and includes many players and some components over which the administrator has limited control. Deep competency in evaluating payer contracts, managing the payment cycle, denials follow-up, appropriate coding of patient encounters, and keeping up with changing payment models are only a few of the key skills required for effective administration of the revenue cycle. In the following chapters, we will see how the revenue cycle fits with the other major competencies for effective financial management of the medical practice.

Notes

1. American Medical Association, *CPT 2015 Professional Edition* (Chicago: American Medical Association, 2014).

2. "NCCI Coding Edits," Centers for Medicare & Medicaid Services, last modified March 2, 2015, www.cms.gov/Medicare/Coding/National CorrectCodInitEd/ NCCICodingEdits.html.

3. Laura Scofea, "The Development and Growth of Employer Provided Health Insurance," *Monthly Labor Review* (March 1994): 3–10, www.bls.gov/OPUB/ MLR/1994/03/art1full.pdf.

4. Scofea, "The Development and Growth of Employer Provided Health Insurance."

5. "About Blue Cross Blue Shield," Blue Cross Blue Shield Association, 2019, www. bcbs.com/abouttheassociation/.

6. Scofea, "The Development and Growth of Employer Provided Health Insurance."

7. "History," Centers for Medicare & Medicaid Services, last modified June 13, 2013, www.cms.gov/AboutCMS/AgencyInformation/History/index.html?redirect=/history/.

8. "Medicare Advantage Fact Sheet," Henry J. Kaiser Family Foundation, May 1, 2014, http://kff.org/medicare/factsheet/medicareadvantagefactsheet/.

9. "Medicaid: A Timeline of Key Developments," Henry J. Kaiser Family Foundation, https://kaiserfamilyfoundation.files.wordpress.com/2008/04/50213 medicaidtimeline.pdf.

10. "Resource Based Relative Value Scale (RBRVS)," Blue Cross and Blue Shield of Alabama, Sept. 2, 2009, www.bcbsal.org/providers/newpaymentmethod ology/RBRVSEducation.pdf.

11. "Sustainable Growth Rate (SGR)," American College of Physicians (ACP), www.acponline.org/advocacy/state_health_policy/hottopics/sgr.pdf.

12. "Physician Quality Reporting System (PQRS)," American Academy of Orthopaedic Surgeons/American Association of Orthopaedic Surgeons (AAOS), www.aaos.org/research/committee/evidence/pqri_intro.asp.

13. Lawrence Wolper, *Physician Practice Management: Essential Operational and Financial Knowledge*, 2nd ed. (Burlington, MA: Jones & Bartlett Learning, 2012), 314.

14. Wolper, *Physician Practice Management*, 332.

15. "Health & Nutrition: Medicare, Medicaid," United States Census Bureau, last modified May 28, 2014, www.census.gov/compendia/statab/cats/ health_nutrition/medicare_medicaid.html.

16. "HEDIS˚ and Quality Compass˚," National Committee for Quality Assurance (NCQA), www.ncqa.org/HEDISQualityMeasurement/ WhatisHEDIS.aspx.

17. "About The Joint Commission," The Joint Commission, 2015, www.joint commission.org/about_us/about_the_joint_commission_main.aspx.

18. Deborah Walker Keegan and Elizabeth W. Woodcock, *The Physician Billing Process: 12 Potholes to Avoid on the Road to Getting Paid*, 3nd ed. (Englewood, CO: Medical Group Management Association, 2016), 85–89.

19. Walker Keegan and Woodcock., *The Physician Billing Process*, 67.

20. Walker Keegan and Woodcock, *The Physician Billing Process*, 102.

21. "Health Information Privacy: HIPAA Administrative Simplification Statute and Rules," U.S. Department of Health and Human Services, www.hhs.gov/ocr/privacy/hipaa/administrative/.

Chapter 2

Managing Cash Flows

One of the most valuable assets a medical group has is cash. Cash provides the means to acquire resources to conduct the practice, satisfy creditors and suppliers of resources, and compensate physicians and staff. Without adequate amounts of cash, the practice would be unable to operate or would experience great hardship and stress. Thus managing cash becomes a matter of continuous focus for the financial manager. The key knowledge and skills necessary to effectively manage cash include managing accounts receivable, anticipating fluctuations impacting cash flow, and analyzing and reporting of cash flow projections.

Cash management should be viewed as a before-the-fact control system. Unlike profit planning, in which operations can continue for a time if losses occur, when a medical group's cash is exhausted, immediate action must take place. By continually planning for cash needs, the group can be certain that adequate cash is available when needed, but excess cash is not accumulated.

Managing the Current Cash Position

There are two important questions the financial manager needs to know: How much cash is available, and where is it held? Ideally the manager should have an accurate picture of both the amount and the timing of cash flows for the entire practice. As we will see later, the cash budget projects cash inflows and cash outflows by month for the next year. An annual picture of cash flows by month shows seasonal patterns and allows the manager to schedule once-a-year payments as well as other discretionary payments, such as capital expenditures and professional liability insurance premiums, during months that are most beneficial. Also, the cash budget may indicate that cash inflows for a particular month will exceed cash outflows. Thus, for that month, the group should have no cash flow problems. However, in other months, cash outflows may be greater than cash inflows, causing a deficit unless a large balance of cash is maintained. Cash planning for the entire year is accomplished through the cash budget, which is covered in a later section. The day-to-day control of cash requires two major tools: the short-term cash plan and the daily cash report.

The Short-Term Cash Plan

The short-term cash plan is a dynamic tool for short-term cash management. The period covered by the plan and the detail of projection depend on the fluctuations of cash and the precision with which the cash is managed. Generally its length is at least one month.

For most medical groups, cash flow projections by day for the next week, and then by week for the remainder of the month, provide an adequate approach to managing short-term cash. For example, the short-term cash plan presents four weeks of data showing daily cash flows for week 1 and weekly cash flows for weeks 2, 3, and 4. At the end of each week, the short-term cash plan is *rolled over*. A new short-term cash plan will show the expected cash flows for week 2 on a daily basis and show the expected cash flows for weeks 3, 4, and 5 on a weekly basis. This arrangement continually rolls over each week, thereby keeping the short-term cash plan current.

The advantages of this short-term cash planning can be illustrated in the following example that uses data in Exhibits 2.1 and 2.2. The short-term cash forecast, as shown in Exhibit 2.1 for the month of January, is prepared based on the organization's longer-term cash budget (covered later). The forecast indicates that there will be a cash

Exhibit 2.1

Short-Term Cash Forecast by Week for the Month of January[1]

	Week 1	Week 2	Week 3	Week 4
Beginning Cash Balance	**$100,000**	**($63,700)**	**($30,500)**	**$10,300**
Cash Inflows				
Electronic payments				
Blue Cross	20,000	20,000	25,000	25,000
Medicare	12,000	12,000	15,000	15,000
Other	15,000	15,000	12,000	12,000
Total Electronic Payments	47,000	47,000	52,000	52,000
Lockbox payments	5,000	7,000	7,000	8,000
Patient payments (front desk)	2,000	2,500	2,500	2,500
Credit card payments	2,000	2,000	2,000	2,000
Capitation payment from HMO	—	20,000	—	—
Other	2,000	1,000	1,500	500
Total Cash Inflows	58,000	79,500	65,000	65,000
Cash Outflows				
Net payroll (including physicians)	—	20,000	—	90,000
Payroll taxes	80,000	—	7,000	—
Refunds	700	800	700	800
Accounts payable	140,000	25,000	15,000	10,000
Other	1,000	500	1,500	250
Total Outflows	221,700	46,300	24,200	101,050
Ending Cash Balance	($63,700)	($30,500)	$10,300	($25,750)

drain in January because of low production in December that will cause low collections in January. Also during January, professional liability insurance premiums will be due and a higher level of production is anticipated, thereby resulting in larger cash outflows.

For simplicity, Exhibit 2.1 presents the tentative short-term cash forecast for the first four weeks limited to weekly cash flows. As can be

Exhibit 2.2

Short-Term Cash Plan by Week for the Month of January[2]

Beginning Cash Balance	Week 1	Week 2	Week 3	Week 4
	$100,000	$26,300	$25,500	$66,300
Cash Inflows				
Electronic payments				
Blue Cross	20,000	20,000	25,000	25,000
Medicare	12,000	12,000	15,000	15,000
Other	15,000	15,000	12,000	12,000
Total Electronic Payments	47,000	47,000	52,000	52,000
Lockbox payments	5,000	7,000	7,000	8,000
Patient payments (front desk)	2,000	2,500	2,500	2,500
Credit card payments	2,000	2,000	2,000	2,000
Capitation payment (HMO)	—	20,000	—	—
Other	2,000	1,000	1,500	500
Sale of investments	40,000	—	—	—
Borrowing	50,000	—	—	—
Total Cash Inflows	148,000	79,500	65,000	65,000
Cash Outflows				
Net payroll (including physicians)	—	20,000	—	90,000
Payroll taxes	80,000	—	7,000	—
Accounts payable	140,000	25,000	15,000	10,000
Refunds	700	800	700	800
Other	1,000	500	1,500	250
Repay borrowing	—	34,000	—	5,000
Total Outflows	221,700	80,300	24,200	106,050
Ending Cash Balance	$26,300	$25,500	$66,300	$25,250

observed, a large cash deficiency appears in the first week of January, primarily because of the payment of the professional liability insurance (included in the $140,000 accounts payable amount). A smaller deficiency occurs in weeks 2 and 4. Assuming the financial manager used sound cash management practices prior to January, the long-term planning of the cash budget would have forced the accumulation of some funds in anticipation of the January deficiencies. Therefore, let us assume that funds generated in earlier months were invested in marketable securities and that a line of credit was established at the bank. Given this tentative short-term forecast in Exhibit 2.1, the financial manager must revise the forecast to meet the cash needs and provide for a minimum cash balance.

A short-term cash plan is developed from the information now available and is shown in Exhibit 2.2. The cash plan is based on a minimum required cash balance of $25,000. Management decided to sell $40,000 of marketable securities and to borrow $50,000 on the line of credit. They planned to repay the loan in the second and fourth weeks as cash was generated. An alternative approach would have been to spread the payment to the insurance company over several months. The choice also must depend on the relative cost of each. In this illustration, the final short-term cash plan met the group's cash needs and maintained a minimum cash balance of $25,000. Note that the short-term cash plan projected cash flows by week for the next month.

Daily projections for weeks 1 and 3 may have indicated the need for additional borrowings if cash payments were scheduled early in the week and cash receipts were expected late in the week.

The Daily Cash Report

A vital report for every medical group is the daily cash report. It acts like the fuel gauge on a car. This report permits the financial member to monitor the cash position on a current basis and to see that the projection in the short-term cash plan is achieved.

Deviations from the short-term cash plan may require corrective action — sometimes immediately. For example, it may be necessary to shift cash from one bank to another, sell or purchase short-term investments, or borrow or repay loans from the line of credit.

The daily cash report is even more important for the group that does not prepare a formal cash budget or a short-term cash plan. Because cash management is carried out informally in those cases, the daily cash report serves as the only tool to plan for cash needs and to monitor the cash position. Exhibit 2.3 illustrates the daily cash report. The key information includes:

- Book and bank balance of each cash account;
- Summary of daily receipts; and
- Summary of daily disbursements.

Some groups may desire only the information on account balances presented at the bottom of Exhibit 2.3. In addition to book (or checkbook) balances, the bank balance may be obtained using internet or telephone banking. This information serves at least two purposes: (1) determining the float position of each account and (2) determining the adequacy of compensating balances. *Float* refers to the lag period from when a check is issued to the time when the check clears the issuer's checking account. *Compensating balances* are additional requirements imposed on borrowers by commercial banks beyond interest charges and require the borrower to maintain a specified demand deposit balance at that bank. Inadequate compensating balances may result in additional service charges, difficulty in obtaining loans, or higher interest rates.

The information in the upper portion of Exhibit 2.3 displays cash collections by pay type and major expenses by category. It is considered good financial management to collect patient payments at the time of service, at least copayment amounts. Note that the illustration provides a line for cash receipts collected at the front desk.

Groups that do not maintain a cash budget or short-term cash plan might include a section on the report providing a cash forecast for the next few days. Financial managers are strongly encouraged to use daily cash reports because they improve cash planning by helping to avert cash crises and allow a more even distribution of cash to physicians. If

Exhibit 2.3

Illustration of Daily Cash Report[3]

Beginning Cash Balance	$_____	
Cash Receipts		
Electronic payments	$_____	
Blue Cross	_____	
Medicare	_____	
Other	_____	
Total Electronic Payments	_____	
Lockbox payments	_____	
Patient payments (front desk)	_____	
Credit card payments	_____	
Capitation payment from HMO	_____	
Other	_____	
Total Cash Receipts	$_____	
Total receipts and beginning balance	$_____	
Cash Disbursements		
Net payroll (including physicians)	$_____	
Payroll taxes	_____	
Accounts payable	_____	
Employer retirement plan contributions	_____	
Refunds	_____	
Other	_____	
Total Disbursements	$_____	
Ending Daily Cash Balance	$_____	

Bank Account/Number	Book Balance	Bank Balance
General account	$_____	$_____
Payroll account	_____	_____
Refunds account	_____	_____
Other	_____	_____
Total Ending Cash Balance	$_____	$_____

Exhibit 2.4
Month-to-Date Cash Spreadsheet for Bank Account[4]

		CASH RECEIPTS					
	Date	Electronic	Lockbox	Credit Card	Clinic	Other	Description
Balance Forward							
Sat	1-Jan						
Sun	2-Jan						
Mon	3-Jan	2,134.76	1,788.22	1,560.22	3,100.00		
Tues	4-Jan	8,977.53	1,020.21	900.00	1,200.00		
Wed	5-Jan	35,000.03	3,901.22	888.22	2,050.00		
Thurs	6-Jan	18,009.22	2,277.53	500.00	4,977.22		
Fri	7-Jan	7,877.24	1,090.43	1,088.88	2,197.90		
Sat	8-Jan						
Sun	9-Jan						
Mon	10-Jan	6,902.12	3,338.97	1,500.00	3,665.00	35,982.11	Capitation HMO
Tues	11-Jan	9,092.71	1,088.66	2,200.00	1,400.22		
Wed	12-Jan	28,799.53	2,398.67	786.44	1,909.50		
Thurs	13-Jan	21,222.34	1,986.46	3,126.33	2,110.30		
Fri	14-Jan	5,877.22	2,238.95	701.00	529.90		
Sat	15-Jan						
Sun	16-Jan						
Mon	17-Jan	4,992.11	1,000.87	210.00	4,201.98		
Tues	18-Jan	9,223.44	2,187.60	890.00	1,602.10		
Wed	19-Jan	37,188.29	1,876.54	3,011.11	1,876.36	3,500.00	Expert Witness Fees
Thurs	20-Jan	23,111.21	2,198.07	1,790.50	2,367.92		
Fri	21-Jan	6,266.59	1,287.45	1,112.55	891.50		
Sat	22-Jan						
Sun	23-Jan						
Mon	24-Jan	6,999.22	977.62	765.00	3,523.67		
Tues	25-Jan	8,902.34	1,238.70	1,890.33	1,785.60		
Wed	26-Jan	39,555.32	2,654.81	3,123.09	3,793.19	79.20	Vendor Refund
Thurs	27-Jan	19,014.23	901.00	888.21	2,054.73		
Fri	28-Jan	8,921.85	3,198.54	791.31	650.34		
Sat	29-Jan						
Sun	30-Jan	5,899.21	2,111.89	810.20	4,590.21		
Mon	31-Jan	12,900.24	1,004.55	1,400.77	1,543.28		
Total		326,866.75	41,766.96	29,934.16	52,020.92	39,561.31	
Total Fee-for-Service Collections						450,588.79	
Total Cash Receipts						490,150.10	

Checks	Tax Deposits	Other	Description	Book Balance	Bank Balance
				167,205.32	306,230.75
				167,205.32	306,230.75
				167,205.32	306,230.75
	119,325.22			56,463.30	73,456.32
59,222.61				9,338.43	65,230.65
				51,177.90	80,230.21
				76,941.87	83,222.31
				89,196.32	92,123.44
				89,196.32	92,123.44
				89,196.32	92,123.44
				140,584.52	141,622.52
15,204.79				139,161.32	152,802.55
				173,055.46	181,203.55
				201,500.89	206,222.52
		83,555.76	Net Payroll	127,292.20	165,222.50
				127,292.20	165,222.50
				127,292.20	165,222.50
				137,697.16	145,930.25
32,627.96				118,972.34	155,222.93
	36,902.44			129,522.20	135,202.22
				158,989.90	162,555.91
				168,547.99	170,987.56
				168,547.99	170,987.56
				168,547.99	170,987.56
19,345.67				161,467.83	180,203.57
				175,284.80	189,202.57
				224,490.41	236,502.66
				247,348.58	249,631.52
	382.01	3,457.82	Refunds	257,070.79	261,305.99
				257,070.79	261,305.99
				270,482.30	272,381.29
	15,982.52	85,201.55	Net Payroll	186,147.07	230,222.91
126,401.03	172,592.19	172,215.13			

administrators believe they do not need to plan for cash needs, they are probably maintaining too much cash. Using daily cash forecasts will frequently lead to a lower financing cost for operations, a stronger credit standing, and more satisfied physicians.

The administrator may find it useful to keep a month-to-date cash spreadsheet, which details the receipts, disbursements, transfers, and running balance by bank account by day for each month (Exhibit 2.4). The information in this spreadsheet can be used to provide a proof of cash for use in connection with the bank reconciliation.

Improving Cash Flows

Medical practices can improve their cash flows in a number of ways, including those outlined in the following sections.

Maintaining a Healthy Revenue Cycle

Effective revenue cycle management will speed up cash flows and spread cash collections more evenly. The revenue cycle is discussed in detail in Chapter 1, but here are more tips:

- Practice personnel should attempt to collect all copayments from patients at the time of service. If practice personnel can compute the amount due after the patient's insurance company pays, the practice should attempt to collect this amount as well.
- Practice management should consider a policy requiring self-pay patients to pay at the time of service and be prepared to work out suitable payment plans for patients who cannot pay larger bills at this time. The practice should communicate the fact that these payments are due at the time of service in advance of the patient's appointment.
- Accepting credit cards makes paying easier for many patients. Also, many health savings plans provide healthcare credit cards for employees to use for their medical bills. These patients can become upset when the

practice does not accept these cards, as they must then complete and turn in the paperwork and wait for their reimbursement.

- Insurance companies should be billed promptly, with special care taken to ensure that the practice is sending a *clean claim*. Denials should be worked promptly. Billing and collection personnel should follow up on unpaid claims from both insurance companies and patients.

Timing of Billing by Suppliers

The practice should strive to time the due dates for its vendor bills to correlate with its cash receipts. For example, a practice that receives a large capitation payment from a health maintenance organization (HMO) during the second week of each month might attempt to arrange for certain vendors' bills to be due after this time. Many suppliers will cooperate in setting more convenient payment dates. Thus financial managers might request that suppliers invoice the group at dates that fit the group's cash flow schedule.

Payment of Vendors

In general, the best practice is to pay bills at the time they are due. If a practice pays its bills early, then it loses the cash flow advantages of using the money for the extra time period. If a practice pays its bills late, then it risks a poor credit rating.

Harvey Mackay, author of *Swim with the Sharks without Being Eaten Alive,* offers a contrarian view on the prompt payment of bills. He advocates paying promptly, claiming that the goodwill this creates with vendors is more valuable than the use of the money for the extra time period. Mackay explains, "The way you pay your bills says something about the kind of person you are to deal with. Whether it's the man who painted your house or the firm that delivers your raw stock, you'll always get a better shake if you pay the same day you get the bill."[5]

Thus managers should weigh the advantage of longer use of funds by waiting until the due date to pay bills against the benefits of maintaining a more favorable relationship with vendors by paying early.

Payment at the End of Discount Periods

When a vendor offers a discount period, the best strategy calls for paying at the end of the discount period. The practice should almost always take advantage of discounts, as missing a discount results in the group paying a higher effective interest rate. For example, if a vendor offers a cash discount of "2/10, net 30," this means that either (1) a 2 percent discount can be taken if paid in 10 days, or, if not, (2) the full amount is due in 30 days. Failing to take advantage of this discount would cost the medical group 2 percent for use of the supplier's money for an additional 20 days. Since there are eighteen 20-day periods in a year, the effective annual rate is approximately 36.5 percent.

Arranging Deferred Financing

Through negotiations with suppliers, it is often possible to make major purchases and extend payments over several months. This is particularly true if the practice is a valuable customer or if the vendor has significant competition. Many suppliers will extend payments for 90 to 120 days without additional cost. In other cases, the added interest a supplier may charge is often lower than the group's borrowing cost.

Controlling Claims Payments

Medical groups that pay claims to other providers, such as those in sub-capitation arrangements, should establish a schedule for paying claims to those providers, for example, paying these claims once or twice a month on set dates. Having a schedule helps the practices keep cash levels high as long as possible and earn income on short-term investments. The desire to control claims payments to the maximum extent must be balanced by any need for favorable relations with physicians and other providers outside the group.

Arranging for Earlier Receipt of Capitation Fees

The practice should attempt to arrange earlier due dates for capitation payments as part of the group's negotiation with the HMO. The HMO itself is normally paid by employer groups in the first half of the month.

Strategic Timing of Payroll

Another strategy is to set the practice's payroll dates to maximize cash flow. For example, because physician payroll is usually a practice's largest expense, it might make sense to pay this at the end of the month. Support staff salaries are often paid semimonthly or biweekly to accommodate those employees' personal budget needs.

Take care in determining the physicians' regular salary (which they expect to receive no matter what) in relationship to their bonus. If the practice sets the regular physician compensation too high, it risks a cash crunch should the practice fail to realize sufficient profits or cash flow. Use regular salary amounts that are easily obtainable but sufficient to meet the physicians' normal living expenses, leaving the bonus pool for excess funds. The timing of bonuses is crucial. For example, a practice with a lower cash flow during the first quarter will probably not want to pay a physician bonus at that time. Cash basis practices will want to pay a bonus at the end of the year for tax-planning purposes.

Managing the Payment of Employer Retirement Plan Contributions

Federal tax laws currently let all employers (including cash basis taxpayers) deduct contributions paid to qualified retirement plans up to the due date of their income tax return (including extensions). For example, a corporate calendar-year practice could wait until its tax return due date of March 15 of the following year to make its retirement plan contribution (or until September 15 if it gets an extension). This deferral can be especially useful to cash basis practices in their attempt to minimize income taxes at the end of the year while maintaining sufficient cash for operations at the beginning of the following year. Be careful not to abuse this tool by pushing contributions too far back while failing to accumulate the cash necessary to fund the contributions; this can create significant cash flow problems when the practice is up against its extended due date and does not have sufficient funds to pay its retirement plan contributions.

Keep in mind that this option to defer retirement plan funding until the tax return due date is only available for the *employer* retirement plan contributions. Amounts withheld from employees for 401(k) deferral contributions or plan loan repayments must be remitted to the plan promptly.

Measuring Cash Flows Using the Cash Flow Statement

Under the accrual method of accounting, the balance sheet (which provides the status of the group's assets, liabilities, and owners' equity) and the income statement (which summarizes the results of operations) present a limited picture of the medical group's financial activities. Comparative balance sheets show the net changes in assets and liabilities but do not reflect the major transactions that brought about these changes. The accrual income statement provides a realistic picture as to the success of practice operations for a given time period but falls short of showing what effect operations have on the cash balance of the practice and what other transactions were undertaken that did not affect the period's revenues and expenses. Thus neither statement provides a full indication of the resources provided and the uses to which they were put during the period. The missing link is to have a presentation of what occurred to perhaps the most vital resource of the group, which is cash. The cash flow statement is directed at presenting this past history for the last accounting period, usually a year.

This discussion of the cash flow statement assumes that the group is following the accrual basis of accounting. A cash flow statement is not required for practices using the cash method of accounting or some other comprehensive basis of accounting. Groups using these other methods may wish to prepare a cash flow statement, particularly if they have large differences between net income and cash flow.

Purposes and Uses of the Cash Flow Statement

Even though we have stressed the importance of the income statement as a crucial measurement of progress in business, many individuals believe that cash flow information is equally important in assessing a business's future performance. The usefulness of the cash flow statement is borne out by its portrayal of information about:

- A practice's activities in generating cash through its major operations or *reason for being*;
- The likelihood and amount of cash distributions to the owner physician and for other reinvestment purposes;
- Its financing activities, including both debt and additional investment by the physicians; and
- Its investing activities, such as the purchase of new equipment or other healthcare practices or entities.

The information on the cash flow statement can assist users or readers of the statement in assessing several factors about the practice, such as its financial and operating risks, its financial flexibility, its liquidity position, and the likelihood of profitability. Each of these factors will be discussed next.

Financial Risk

Financial risk involves the likelihood that the practice's cash flows may become inadequate to cover its debt service requirements (assuming there is debt owed by the group), that is, that cash will be insufficient to cover periodic debt interest and principal payments. Financial risk is a function of the group's financial structure (relative proportions of debt and equity), meaning the lower the portion of debt to equity, the smaller the financial risk. Because debt repayment and interest requirements are satisfied by cash payments, which are provided largely from operational earnings, information about the group's cash flows from operations is useful in assessing its ability to cover the debt service requirements. A greater ability to cover these requirements results in a lower financial risk.

Operating Risk

Operating risk involves the likelihood of a practice experiencing unexpected reductions in the demand for its services. If this risk is high, cash flows from operations may become insufficient to provide funds to continue the practice at its normal level. It may become necessary to obtain cash from outside the group or have physician-owners contribute additional funds. The availability, amount, and timing of these needed funds may place a serious burden on the group's financial position and operating capability.

Financial Flexibility

Financial flexibility is related to operating risk and encompasses the ability of a business to weather bad times and respond to new investment opportunities as they come along. For example, the severity of a high level of operating risk can be alleviated if the practice can borrow funds or sell unneeded assets. Also, by having funds readily accessible to invest in a new piece of equipment or a new service line, the group may be able to increase its cash flow from operations fairly quickly. The reporting of the cash flows from operations thus shows the group's sensitivity to situations that may require immediate cash.

Liquidity

Liquidity refers to the makeup of the current assets and the proportion of those assets that are comprised of cash and near-term cash items, such as highly marketable securities. The more liquid a group is, the less chance it will experience cash flow problems and strains. It will also survive downturns more easily or be able to take advantage of new investment opportunities with available cash. Accurate assessment of a group's liquidity position is important.

Profitability

The cash flow statement helps to show the relationship between accrual net income reported on the income statement and cash flows. Sometimes, a group will show a high level of net income but lack sufficient funds to distribute cash to the physicians or invest in other new options. Identifying the relationships between income and cash flows helps to project meaningful forecasts of earnings and cash flows.

In summary, a cash flow statement provides management and interested outside individuals with information to assess the following:

- Future cash flow potential;
- The means to pay debt service obligations and other liabilities;
- The ability to distribute cash to the physicians;
- Why earnings and net cash receipts and payments differ; and
- Investing and financing transactions.

Further, the cash flow statement can provide answers to some questions frequently heard among physicians about their group's operations, such as:

- Why are cash distributions to physicians less than the net income for the group?
- Where did the group raise additional cash besides the cash flow from operating the practice?
- How are the new acquisitions (e.g., new group just acquired or new equipment) being financed?
- Is the group borrowing funds to continue the distribution of cash to physicians at a certain level?

Elements of the Cash Flow Statement

Cash flow statements must categorize cash flows into three discrete types: operating, investing, and financing. This division emphasizes the relationship among certain components of cash flows that will assist in the analysis of financial performance. By having both cash inflows and cash outflows within each of the three categories, cash flows are perceived as related to each other, such as cash proceeds from borrowing transactions and cash repayments of borrowings shown under the financing category of the statement.

A description of the three categories of activities used in cash flow statements follows. Exhibit 2.5 presents a summary of the major cash inflow and outflow transactions found in the categories within the statement.

Exhibit 2.5

Statement of Cash Flows — Three Categories of Cash Inflows and Outflows[6]

Cash Inflows	Cash Outflows
Operating Activities	
• Cash from patients	• Cash purchases of supplies
• Collection of accounts receivable	• Payment of accounts payable, payroll, and other services
• Receipt of interest, rent, dividends, and other cash revenues	• Payment of interest, rent, and other cash and accrued expenses
Investing Activities	
• Sale of investment securities	• Purchases of investment securities
• Sale of property, plant and equipment, and intangible assets	• Purchases of property, plant and equipment, and intangible assets
• Collections of notes receivable and other loans	• Loans made or purchased
Financing Activities	
• Obtaining short-term or long-term loans	• Repayment of loans
• Issue of capital stock, mortgages, notes, etc.	• Repurchase of capital stock and retirement of bonds and other long-term debts
	• Payment of dividends

Operating Activities

Operating activities are associated with delivering medical services or products to patients as the normal activity of the practice. The cash effects of these activities are the cash inflows (such as collections from patients or third-party payers) and cash outflows (such as payments for supplies and salaries). Generally, most of these transactions wind up as items on the income statement, although their recognition on that statement may differ in timing from that on the cash flow statement because of the accrual cash-basis dichotomy. (See examples in Exhibit 2.5.)

Investing Activities

Investing activities include cash inflows and outflows related to investments, such as purchasing or selling equipment, or buying or selling investment securities. (See examples in Exhibit 2.5.)

Financing Activities

Financing activities pertain to the various aspects of providing financing to the practice, such as obtaining and repaying loans from creditors, receiving additional contributions from physicians as further investment in the practice, and dividends and distributions of retained earnings or capital to physicians and other owners. (See examples in Exhibit 2.5.)

Presentation Format of the Cash Flow Statement

A formal cash flow statement for the East Slope Medical Group is presented in Exhibit 2.6.

To support the underlying sources of the cash flow data, East Slope Medical Group's balance sheet and income statement are also presented in Exhibits 2.7 and 2.8.

Note the major breakdown of the cash flow statement into the three basic segments: operating, investing, and financing. Also observe how the combined changes in these three categories explain the net change in the cash balance (decrease of $40,000) during the year 2015. The beginning balance of cash ($240,000) is added to the net change in cash to produce the ending cash balance ($200,000), which ties out to the cash balance on the balance sheet.

Direct vs. Indirect Method

In preparing the Operating Activities section of the cash flow statement, two choices are available: the direct method and the indirect method. The direct method shows the major types of operating cash receipts, such as cash received from patients, and cash payments, such as cash paid for supplies, salaries, and other services of the practice, to arrive at a net amount of cash provided by operating activities. The indirect method computes the same amount of net cash provided by operating activities but accomplishes it by a circuitous route. The starting point is net income shown on the accrual-based income statement to which several types of other adjustments (summarized

Exhibit 2.6
East Slope Medical Group's Cash Flow Statement[7]

	2015	2014
Cash Flows from Operating Activities		
Net income (loss)	$37,000	$3,000
Depreciation	120,000	70,000
Unrealized gain on marketable security	(15,000)	—
(Gain) on disposal of equipment	(20,000)	—
Unrealized gains and losses on investments	—	—
Deferred income taxes	15,000	(10,000)
Changes in assets and liabilities:		
(Increase) decrease in accounts receivable	(50,000)	42,000
(Increase) in accounts receivable (other)	1,000	(1,000)
(increase) decrease in prepaid expenses	(2,000)	4,000
Increase (decrease) in accounts payable	4,000	(12,000)
Increase (decrease) in payroll, benefits, and taxes payable	9,000	12,000
Increase (decrease) in claims payable	3,000	(4,000)
Increase (decrease) in claims payable IBNR*	1,000	(2,000)
Increase (decrease) in income taxes payable	1,000	(12,000)
Net cash flows from operating activities	104,000	90,000
Cash Flows from Investing Activities		
Purchase of marketable securities	(100,000)	—
Purchase of leasehold improvements	(10,000)	(25,000)
Sale of equipment	20,000	—
Purchase of land for future clinic site	—	—
Purchase of equipment	(345,000)	(23,000)
Net cash flows from investing activities	(435,000)	(48,000)
Cash Flows from Financing Activities		
Net increase (decrease) in notes payable	(95,000)	(25,000)
Net increase in long-term debt	326,000	(55,000)
Proceeds from issuance of common stock	60,000	—
Net cash flows from financing activities	291,000	(80,000)
Increase (decrease) in Cash	(40,000)	(38,000)
Cash at Beginning of Year	240,000	278,000
Cash at End of Year	$200,000	$240,000

* IBNR, incurred but not reported.

Exhibit 2.7
East Slope Medical Group's Balance Sheet[8]

	2015	2014
Assets		
Current Assets:		
Cash	$200,000	$240,000
Marketable securities	115,000	—
Patient accounts receivable, net of allowance for doubtful accounts of $50,000 in 2015 and $47,000 in 2014	640,000	590,000
Accounts receivable — other	2,000	3,000
Deferred tax debits — current	—	—
Prepaid expenses	12,000	10,000
Total current assets	969,000	843,000
Investment:		
Land held for future clinic site	150,000	150,000
Property and equipment, at cost:		
Leasehold improvements	75,000	65,000
Equipment	625,000	575,000
	700,000	640,000
Less: Accumulated Depreciation and Amortization	325,000	500,000
Property and equipment, net	375,000	140,000
Other Assets:		
Goodwill	15,000	15,000
Total Assets	$1,509,000	$1,148,000
Liabilities and Stockholders' Equity		
Current Liabilities:		
Notes payable	$—	$95,000
Current maturities of long-term debt	66,000	—
Accounts payable	60,000	56,000
Accrued payroll, benefits, and taxes	210,000	201,000
Claims payable	16,000	13,000
Claims payable — incurred but not received	3,000	2,000
Income taxes payable	2,000	1,000
Deferred taxes	15,000	5,000
Total current liabilities	372,000	373,000
Long-Term Liabilities:		
Long-term debt, less current maturities	260,000	—
Deferred taxes	15,000	10,000
Total long-term liabilities	275,000	10,000
Total liabilities	647,000	383,000
Stockholders' Equity:		
Common stock, $1 par, authorized 200,000 shares: issued and outstanding 100,000 shares	100,000	90,000
Contributed capital in excess of par	325,000	275,000
Retained earnings	437,000	400,000
Total stockholders' equity	862,000	765,000
Total liabilities and stockholders' equity	$1,509,000	$1,148,000

Exhibit 2.8
East Slope Medical Group's Income Statement[9]

	2015	2014
Revenues		
Patient service revenue (net of contractual allowances and discounts)	$7,100,000	$6,590,000
Provision for bad debts	(100,000)	(90,000)
Net fee-for-service revenue	7,000,000	6,500,000
Capitation revenue, net	200,000	220,000
Other	110,000	90,000
Total medical revenue	7,310,000	6,810,000
Operating Cost		
Support Staff Costs:		
Staff salaries	1,680,000	1,600,000
Payroll taxes	160,000	153,000
Employee benefits	260,000	230,000
Total support staff cost	2,100,000	1,983,000
General Operating Cost		
Information technology	190,000	200,000
Drug supply	250,000	252,000
Medical and surgical supply	170,000	175,000
Depreciation	120,000	70,000
Professional liability insurance	90,000	85,000
Other insurance premiums	11,000	10,500
Building and occupancy	620,000	610,000
Administrative supplies and services	103,000	105,000
Professional and consulting fees	70,000	75,000
Clinical laboratory	260,000	240,000
Radiology and imaging	90,000	80,000
Promotion and marketing	32,000	30,000
Total general operating cost	2,006,000	1,932,500
Total operating cost	4,106,000	3,915,500
Total Medical Revenue after Operating Cost	3,204,000	2,894,500
Less: NPP* Cost	690,000	600,000
Total Medical Revenue after Operating and NPP Cost	2,514,000	2,294,500
Less: Physician Cost	2,350,000	2,200,000
Net Income (Loss) after Provider-Related Expenses	164,000	94,500
Other Income (Expense):		
Interest expense (net)	(150,000)	(90,000)
Unrealized gain on marketable securities	15,000	—
Gain on disposal of equipment	20,000	—
Interest expense (net)	(115,000)	(90,000)
Income before Provision for Income Taxes	49,000	4,500
Provision for (reduction of) Income Taxes	12,000	1,500
Net Income (Loss)	37,000	3,000
Retained Earnings, Beginning of Year	400,000	397,000
Retained Earnings, End of Year	$437,000	$400,000

*NPP, nonphysician provider.

in Exhibit 2.9) are added or deducted. These adjustments include add-backs for noncash expenses such as depreciation, additions or deductions for changes in specific current asset and current liability accounts, and add-backs or deductions for gains and losses incurred from the disposition of long-term assets. While somewhat confusing, the indirect method does present items that explain the differences between accrual income and cash flows from operating activities that are not included in the body of the cash flow statement under the direct method. It is also generally less time consuming for the accountants to prepare, because the numbers primarily come from the income statement and the changes in the balance sheet. Most cash flow statements found in general practice follow the indirect approach.

The following interpretative inferences about the contents of the cash flow statement for the East Slope Medical Group for 2015 in Exhibit 2.6 should be noted:

- The net income ($37,000) on the income statement for the year ended December 31, 2015, is the first item shown under the Operating Activities section that is prepared following the indirect method. Notice that this amount is less than the net cash provided from operating activities ($104,000). This is primarily caused by the noncash expense for depreciation of $120,000 being added back to net income to increase the cash flow from operations. The $50,000 increase in the accounts receivable balance had a negative effect on the net cash provided from operating activities. The practice's total medical revenue for 2015 increased by $500,000, a greater than 7 percent increase over the level achieved in 2014. But part of the increase in revenue was not collected at the end of 2015, as evidenced by the increase in accounts receivable.
- This revelation about the disparity between accrual net income and cash provided by operations shows one of the valued information elements that the cash flow statement makes apparent and might be used as a way to explain (in

- part) why cash distributions to physicians might be less than the corresponding net income.
- Other adjustments to net income in the Operating Activities section of the cash flow statement show the offsetting interplay between the changes in various current asset and current liability accounts, such as the increase in accounts receivable discussed earlier, which decreased cash flow from operations, and the increases in accounts payable and accrued payroll, benefits, and taxes, which have the effect of increasing cash flows from operations.
- Under cash flows from investing activities, we note that the practice purchased marketable securities for $100,000 and equipment with a cost of $345,000. The equipment acquisition was apparently financed by the issuance of a long-term note payable (net of current-year repayments) of $326,000, as indicated under cash flows from financing activities. Note also that short-term notes payable were retired (totaling $95,000) during the period. Also, note that the practice received $60,000 from a new physician shareholder in exchange for the issuance of stock.
- The ending cash balance of $200,000 represents a decrease from the balance of cash at the beginning of the period, which was $240,000. By reviewing the statement of cash flows, we can see the combination of operational and financing cash flows that caused the change in this balance.

Do not confuse the cash flow statement with an income statement prepared using the cash basis. The latter document might be referred to as a statement of cash receipts and disbursements. This statement only reflects cash receipts from patients and other payers for the rendering of medical services, which are considered revenues for the period under the cash basis and shows only cash payments for expenditures classified as expenses to produce the revenue. The cash flow statement shows not only cash flow from operations but also cash inflows and outflows for other transactions not shown on the statement of cash receipts and disbursements, such as proceeds and repayments of loans, acquisitions of equipment, and other long-term investments. Thus the statement of cash receipts and disbursements is a limited view of cash movements during an accounting period and is not equivalent to a cash flow statement.

Forecasting and Planning Future Cash Flows

Earlier, we introduced the short-term cash plan that predicts cash flows for the immediate future of the group's operations, that is, for several weeks or days within the next month. Its objective is to identify potential cash shortages and excesses so that the financial manager can take appropriate action to manage the current cash position. Now let's turn to planning for a full year.

The Cash Budget

A logical extension of the short-term planning thrust is the cash budget, which schedules the timing of cash flows by month for the coming year. The cash budget represents the major instrument for planning the use of cash during the next operating year. As a planning instrument, it is the result of a deliberate and careful process of scrutinizing the scope and timing of the operations for the following year and measuring the effects of these events on the cash balances needed for carrying out the total group plan. A cash budget is more than a mere prediction of what cash flows will be; it also forecasts cash needs. The cash budget assists in planning future cash flows in these ways:

- Because the final cash budget is the result of a series of trial drafts of cash forecasts, each trial raises questions about whether the operating plans are too ambitious for the cash that will be generated in the next year. If so, some revisions may then be made to the operating plans.
- The cash budget will show when and if a short-term loan is needed and when it can be repaid.
- The cash budget identifies the month that is best for scheduling discretionary or unusual payments, such as bonuses, once-a-year debt service, and annual professional liability insurance premiums.

Exhibit 2.9

Calculating Operating Cash Flow from Net Income (Indirect Method)[10]

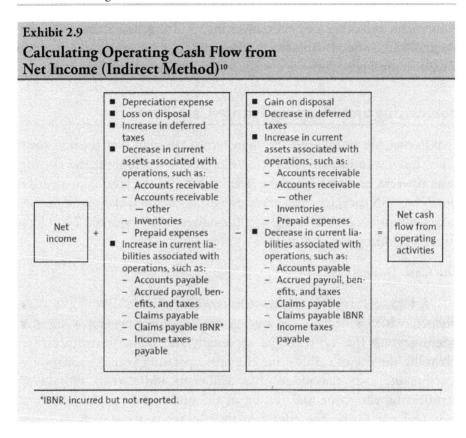

*IBNR, incurred but not reported.

- The cash budget can anticipate the development of a continuing cash surplus that calls for a review of investment possibilities, a reduction of debt, or an additional distribution to the physician-owners.

Clearly, these examples show that the cash budget is a useful tool for internal planning. It can assist management in highlighting key decisions related to cash for the coming year. Also, once adopted, the cash budget may be used as a control benchmark that, when compared with actual cash flows, will indicate the accuracy of cash flow predictions and the need for revising projections for future months.

Another important function of the cash budget is its use in negotiating a loan or line of credit from banks and other lending institutions. A key component of the loan application is the cash budget. Lenders are favorably impressed by cash planning, especially when it is at a level of detail that shows the overall cash picture, along with why the loan is needed and when the loan is likely to be repaid. During periods of tight credit, even preferred borrowers will increasingly be asked to provide cash projections. To volunteer this information in advance is a hallmark of strong overall planning, a sign of good management, and an indication of an intent and ability to repay the loan requested.

The cash budget, like other financial plans, is no better than the sources of data on which is it based. For this reason, we will indicate the data and sources of information needed to construct a cash budget in the next section.

Cash Budget Data and Sources

To build a cash budget for a medical group, the following data is necessary:

- Beginning cash balance;
- Projected cash receipts from patients and third-party payers (also miscellaneous income);
- Projected cash operating expenses;
- Projected cash expenditures for capital acquisitions and long-term investments;
- Projected cash receipts from other sources (e.g., sale of investments);
- Required cash borrowing and debt repayment; and
- Ending cash balance.

This data may be arranged in any format that is useful to the group's management. The format shown in Exhibit 2.10 emphasizes the importance of operations to the cash position. It also highlights, in sequence, the impact of non-operating sources of cash, non-operating uses of cash, and cash borrowings on the ending cash balance. The next section introduces the supporting schedules for this cash budget, along with a discussion about the related data sources.

The Beginning Cash Balance

This balance is the actual amount shown in the accounting records for the beginning cash balance. If the cash budget is prepared before the end of the current year, the beginning cash balance must be estimated.

Projected Cash Receipts from Patients and Third-Party Payers

The key element in the preparation of any budget is the projected volume of service to be provided. This level affects both the cash budget and the profit plan in two ways:

1. The amount of cash to be collected from patients is a direct result of billings for the services performed.

2. The amounts of variable operating expenses (such as supplies) and step-fixed operating expenses (such as many medical support salaries) relate to the level of activity. This factor also has an effect on the relationships among cost, volume of service, and profits.

Several approaches can be used to project the level of services and future revenue. Each of these methods starts with a projection of the volume of services to be provided to patients. For the fee-for-service portion of revenue projection, gross charges are determined by applying the proposed fee schedule to this projected volume of services.

Estimated adjustments must be deducted from gross charges to arrive at billings to patients and third-party payers.

A practical approach to projecting volume of activity involves asking physician and ancillary department heads to forecast the volume of service they expect to provide during the next year. As a starting point, each physician is provided with the actual amount of service (number of patients seen or procedures performed) by month and in total for the year. The physician then indicates the percentage change, above or below last year, for each month and for the year as a whole.

The amount of estimated cash collections by month are determined by applying historical collection patterns to the billings of patients. To illustrate, assume the historical collection pattern is:

- 30 percent collected in the month of billings
- 50 percent collected in the first month after billings
- 10 percent collected in the second month after billings
- 5 percent collected in the third month after billings
- 5 percent uncollectible

If January billings are $200,000, $60,000 for those billings will be collected during January; $100,000 in February; $20,000 in March; and $10,000 in April. In addition, $10,000 will not be collected. Cash collected in January will include 5 percent of October billings, 10 percent of November billings, 50 percent of December billings, and 30 percent of January billings. Exhibit 2.11 illustrates the determination of estimated cash collections by month from estimated patient billings. January billings are $200,000, while collections are $173,000. Billings in February and March are $250,000, while cash collections are $201,000 and $228,500, respectively.

Projected Cash Operating Expenses

Data for the operating expenses in the cash budget can come from three sources:

1. Last year's cash expense data, by month, adjusted for any anticipated changes such as the level of staffing, rates of compensation, and price changes;

2. A consolidation of cash expenses prepared by responsibility centers that relates to their planned level of activity; and

3. A monthly profit plan on a cash basis.

Exhibit 2.12 shows a supporting schedule of cash operating expenses by month. Totals from this schedule are included in the cash budget presented in Exhibit 2.10.

Exhibit 2.10

Cash Budget[11]

Upper Mountain Medical Group
Cash Budget for the Year Ended 12/31/2014

Supporting Schedule Exhibit Number		January	February	March
2.11	Cash collections from patients	$173,000	$201,000	$218,500
2.12	Less cash operating expenses	236,015	170,515	174,515
	Cash increase (decrease) from operations	($63,015)	$30,485	$43,985
	Add beginning balance	14,000	10,000	12,470
	Ending cash balance before nonoperating and financial transactions Add: cash from nonoperating sources	($49,015)	$40,485	$56,455
2.14	Sale of short-term investments	35,000	0	0
	Subtotal	($14,015)	$40,485	$56,455
	Less: cash payments for nonoperating items			
2.15	Payment on installment debt for land	2,000	2,000	2,000
2.15	Repayment of short-term debt	0	26,015	0
2.13	Assets in capital budget	0	0	10,000
2.14	Purchase of short-term investments	0	0	33,000
	Subtotal	$2,000	$28,015	$45,000
2.15	Ending cash balance before borrowing	($16,015)	$12,470	$11,455
	Add: borrowing to maintain minimum cash balance	26,015	0	0
	Ending cash balance	$10,000	$12,470	$11,455

If responsibility centers are identified, their managers should project the amount of operating expenses necessary to support their center's agreed-on level of activities for the next year. After these projections are obtained and approved, they must be translated into cash outlays by month. If the responsibility centers were involved in preparing profit plans, however, the first step in quantifying operating expenses for the following year is already completed.

Exhibit 2.11
Budgeted Cash Collections from Patients[12]

Upper Mountain Medical Group for the Year Ended 12/31/2014

Estimated Patient Billings Related to Budget Year		Estimated Cash Collections by Months in the Budget Year*			
		January	February	March	etc.
October	$200,000	$10,000	$—	$—	$—
November	180,000	18,000	9,000	—	—
		85,000	17,000	8,500	—
December	170,000	60,000	100,000	20,000	10,000
		—	75,000	125,000	25,000
January	200,000	—	—	75,000	125,000
February	250,000				
March	250,000				
	etc.				
Cash Collections		$173,000	$201,000	$228,500	$ etc.

* The assumed collection percentages are as follows:
- 30% collected in the month of billing
- 50% collected in the first month after billing
- 10% in the second month after billing
- 5% in the third month after billing
- 5% uncollectible

Projected Cash Expenditures for Capital Assets and Investments

Capital budgeting relates to prioritizing and evaluating proposals for the acquisition of fixed assets and other long-term investments. The preferred decision rule and techniques require all changes in cash flows caused by a capital asset proposal to be scheduled by future time periods. There are at least three possible effects these cash flows may have on the cash budget:

1. There is usually an initial investment of cash;

2. The net cash inflow generated by the new asset will take the form of increased revenue, decreased operating costs, or a combination of the two; and

3. There may be additional cash receipts from sources, such as borrowings or investments by physician stockholders, used to finance the new asset.

101

In Exhibit 2.10, the $10,000 planned expenditure for the purchase of capital assets was purposely delayed to March when larger cash collections from patients were projected. If the asset had been acquired in January, additional borrowings would have been required. A February acquisition would have required postponement of a portion of the loan repayment to March. Trial cash budgets allow the manager to assess when it is best to acquire a new capital asset in view of other cash flows.

Exhibit 2.13 shows the approved $10,000 outlay that has met all the criteria established by the medical group for acquiring capital assets. In this illustration, there are no acquisitions of long-term investments such as securities or land held for future use. They would be included in this supporting schedule because they require analyses similar to those of operating capital assets.

Projected Cash Receipts from Other Sources

Cash from operations will likely be the medical group's major source of cash. Other sources of cash aside from borrowing might include:

- Sale of investments, including real property no longer used in operations;
- Sale of furniture, fixtures, and equipment no longer used in operations; and
- Cash invested by owners.

The major uses of cash include:

- Acquisition of capital assets and long-term investments;
- Acquisition of short-term investments, such as marketable securities;
- Payment of cash dividends; and
- Other cash distributions to owners besides compensation.

One reason for segregating other sources and uses of cash from both operating cash flows and transactions related to borrowing is because of

Exhibit 2.12
Budgeted Cash Operating Expenses[12]

Upper Mountain Medical Group for the Year Ended 12/31/2014				
	January	February	March	etc.
Human resources expenses				
Physicians' salaries	$77,560	$77,560	$77,560	
Nurses' salaries	21,420	21,420	21,420	
Ancillary department salaries	15,225	15,225	15,225	
Administrative and staff salaries	8,550	8,550	8,550	
Medical support salaries	9,200	9,200	9,200	
Housekeeping and security salaries	1,560	1,560	1,560	
	$133,515	$133,515	$133,515	
Physical resource expenses				
Supplies (detail oriented)	$11,500	$11,500	$11,500	
Occupancy and use — building	9,000	9,000	9,000	
Occupancy and use — utilities	5,000	4,000	4,000	
Maintenance and repairs	2,500	2,500	2,500	
	$28,000	$27,000	$27,000	
Purchased service and general and administrative expenses				
Data processing	$5,000	$5,000	$5,000	
Professional accounting services	0	0	3,000	
Professional liability insurance	65,000	0	0	
General and administrative	$4,500	5,000	6,000	
	$74,500	$10,000	$14,000	
Total cash operating expenses	$236,015	$170,515	$174,515	

their more discretionary nature. Usually, the administration exercises judgment as to which months to include these cash flows.

In Exhibit 2.14, the only source illustrated involves the disposition of short-term investments in January in the amount of $35,000, followed by their virtual replacement in March. A possible alternative available to the financial manager would have been to further increase short-term borrowing in January instead.

Exhibit 2.13
Planned Expenditures for Capital Assets[14]

Upper Mountain Medical Group for the Year Ended 12/31/2014

	January	February	March	etc.
Planned purchase of capital assets				
Compact automobile	$0	0	$6,000	
Waiting room furniture	0	0	4,000	
Totals	$0	$0	$10,000	
Planned purchase of investments				
Land held for future use	$0	$0	$0	
Totals	$0	$0	$10,000	

Perhaps by using these short-term investments as security for the loan, its cost could have been reduced, and the transaction costs on the sale and later repurchase of the short-term investments could have been avoided.

Borrowing Cash and Debt Repayment

Borrowing for periods of a year or less is called *short term*. Banks may require such loans to be "cleaned up" once a year before any further short-term credit is granted. When cash is borrowed on a short-term basis, it should provide financing for seasonal needs. If not repaid out of operations within a year, it must be replaced by a more permanent source. Term or installment loans range from 1 to 5 years and sometimes as long as 10. They are commonly used to finance equipment acquisitions that should generate additional cash flows above the required debt service. Long-term loans, in excess of 5 to 10 years, are usually related to financing improved real property that will generate sufficient cash flows beyond insurance, repairs, taxes, and so on to cover their debt service.

Leases are a hybrid type of debt financing. They vary from month-to-month; arrangements at one extreme to an installment purchase at the other. As with other borrowing, the cash flows generated by the leased asset should sustain the lease payments called for by the agreement.

104

Exhibit 2.14
Planned Other Sources and Uses of Cash[15]

Upper Mountain Medical Group for the Year Ended 12/31/2014

	January	February	March	etc.
Planned other sources				
Sale of short-term investments	$35,000	0	$0	
Sale of real property	0	0	0	
Investments by owners	0	0	0	
Totals	$35,000	$0	$0	
Planned other uses				
Purchase of short-term investments	$0	$0	$33,000	
Payment of dividends	0	0	0	
Totals	$0	$0	$33,000	

Inattention to loan terms can lead to severe financial problems. For example, a 5-year loan is used to finance an asset having a 10-year payback period. In this instance, the trial cash budget, if realistically prepared, should provide a warning signal to management. With increased debt service, a chronic cash drain will appear, indicating a need for either longer term financing or reduced expansion plans.

As shown in Exhibit 2.15, the use of a short-term loan is needed because the payment of the professional liability insurance for the medical group causes a severe cash drain in January. The cash budget also shows that this loan can be repaid in February according to the projected other cash needs and sources. Although it could be easily argued that this loan should be for a longer period, because it is financing insurance that will benefit the entire year, it makes sense to pay it off in February and save interest. The loan has also been cleaned up, which sets the stage for another loan should it be needed later in the year.

The other loan repayment included in Exhibit 2.15 is the result of an investment decision in a prior period. The medical group is paying for this land at the agreed-on rate of $2,000 per month.

Exhibit 2.15
Planned Borrowing and Debt Payment[16]

Upper Mountain Medical Group for the Year Ended 12/31/2014

	January	February	March	etc.
Planned borrowing				
Short-term loan	$26,015	$0	$0	
Totals	$26,015	$0	$0	
Planned debt repayment				
Short-term loan	$0	$26,015	$0	
Installment debt for land	2,000	2,000	2,000	
Totals	$2,000	$28,015	$2,000	

Ending Cash Balance

Turning back to Exhibit 2.10, one can see that "ending cash balance" is used within captions at three points in the cash budget. The first shows the amount of cash that would result from adding planned cash flows from operations to the beginning cash balance. This number helps the financial manager decide on the month in which to include discretionary sources and/or uses of cash. In a similar manner, the line captioned "ending cash balance before borrowing," shows what amount, if any, must be borrowed to maintain a minimum balance. The final ending cash balance is the projected position of cash at the end of the month after taking all planned cash transactions as well as the beginning cash balance into account. This figure would be used in the projected balance sheet if one were prepared.

Keeping the Cash Budget Updated

The cash budget should be maintained a year in advance by adding three more months at the end of each completed quarter. Within the quarter, a monthly short-term cash forecast is prepared using the best current data available.

As mentioned earlier, the short-term forecast is broken down by weeks to facilitate cash management of the current position. If the cash budget varies widely from actual data, it will be necessary to revise the budget completely at the end of the quarter.

Summary

At various points in this section, we noted the interrelationship between the operating plan (profit plan) and the cash budget. Amounts derived from the profit plan, such as receipts from patients and cash operating expenses, are key elements in the cash budget. Acquisition of, or changes in, the assets and their finance (resource plans) are also necessary to complete the budget.

It is not surprising that the cash budget is often called a *residual budget* because it is the result of all other financial plans; however, this should not lead anyone to the conclusion that the cash budget is no more than a carryover total. It is much more, particularly in the trial cash budget stage. At that point, it identifies the temporary excesses or surpluses of cash that call for investment or borrowing plans. It diagnoses chronic cash drains in advance, which will call for a change in the scope of plans and/or additional permanent financing. It also provides guidance for shifting discretionary cash receipts or payments to an appropriate month.

Exhibit 2.16 shows the importance of the cash budget in coordinating both operating plans and resource plans. Finally, it is a strong managerial tool for negotiating needed financing.

Internal Cash Controls

Because cash is such a volatile asset, internal control over it must be strong, continuous, and all encompassing. The major approaches to ensuring that controls are effective are covered in Chapter 6 of this volume.

Exhibit 2.16
Cash Budget Coordination[17]

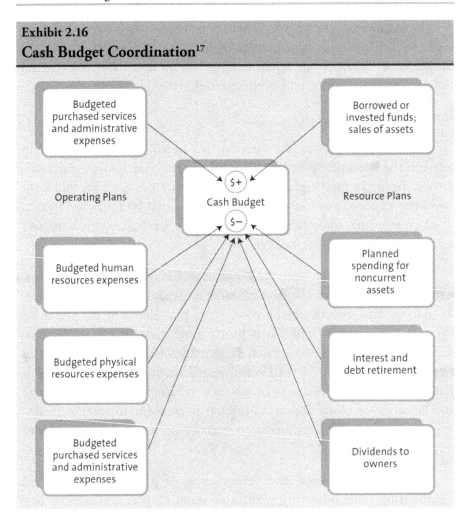

Managing Short-Term Investments

Assets that are closely related to cash are the short-term investments that medical groups enter into for short periods of time. When the cash position is being built up to meet a large planned expenditure later in the year, the cash in excess of normal needs should be invested for a return. These temporary excesses in the cash account can be transferred to the group's savings account or into other short-term investments and then returned to cash when needed later.

The most frequently mentioned types of investments that groups select are savings accounts, certificates of deposit, U.S. Treasury bills and notes, money market mutual funds, and commercial paper. Some of these investment instruments may need explanation:

- *Savings accounts* are comprised of time deposits and passbook savings accounts with banks. They earn a fixed interest rate.

- *Certificates of deposit* (or CDs) are marketable receipts for funds that have been deposited in a bank for a fixed period of time and earn a fixed interest rate. Certificates are offered by banks in a variety of denominations and range in maturity from one month to several years.

- *U.S. Treasury bills* are perhaps the most popular short-term investment vehicle. A Treasury bill is a direct obligation of the U.S. government sold on a regular basis by the U.S. Treasury in denominations of $10,000 and upward to $1 million. Maturities are one month, three months, six months, and one year. Interest rates vary depending on the short-term money market conditions.

- *Money market mutual funds*, sometimes called *liquid-asset funds*, sell their shares to raise cash, and by pooling the funds of large numbers of small savers, they build their liquid-asset portfolios. Investors can start their accounts with as little as $1,000 and use these as an investment outlet for small amounts of excess cash. Withdrawals can be made quickly from these accounts using checks drawn on the account balance.

- Commercial paper represents unsecured, short-term negotiable promissory notes issued by large, well-established companies that need funds for a short time period. Denominations are usually in fairly large sums ($100,000) and thus, would probably be sought primarily by larger medical groups as an investment medium.

The primary characteristics of these investment options are their short-term maturity dates and the ability for the investors to convert them back into cash with a minimum of effort and with less risk of losing their original investment amount. Thus financial managers must be careful in selecting short-term investments, as safety of principal is the paramount concern.

To incorporate any short-term investments into the cash management process, it is important that these investments are monitored and the amounts of their current values are developed when these investment balances are needed for planning purposes. Thus each investment should be listed on a schedule that includes this information:

- Current market value;
- Purchase and maturity date (if applicable);
- Income to date; and
- Yield percentage.

Also, the total investment balances for the current and previous months should be made available. This information can be used in preparing short-term cash forecasts if investments are to be liquidated within the month. If they are not, their proceeds should be included in the cash budget for the month in which they are liquidated.

Conclusion

Cash management is a key component of a medical practice's financial infrastructure. A successful practice must be able to meet its current financial obligations at any given point in time. The effective administrator manages the day-to-day flows of cash in and out of the practice as well as monitoring internal controls over cash processes and reporting the current and projected cash position of the practice.

Notes

1. From *Financial Management for Medical Groups: A Resource for New and Experienced Managers*, 3rd ed. (Englewood, CO: MGMA, 2014), 222, exhibit 8.1.

2. From *Financial Management for Medical Groups*, 223, exhibit 8.2.

3. From *Financial Management for Medical Groups*, 225, exhibit 8.3.

4. From *Financial Management for Medical Groups*, 226, exhibit 8.4.

5. Harvey B. Mackay, *Swim with the Sharks without Being Eaten Alive: Outsell, Outmanage, Outmotivate, and Outnegotiate Your Competition* (New York: HarperCollins, 2005), 124.

6. From *Financial Management for Medical Groups*, 241, exhibit 8.10.

7. From *Financial Management for Medical Groups*, 243, exhibit 8.11.

8. From *Financial Management for Medical Groups*, 244, exhibit 8.12.

9. From *Financial Management for Medical Groups*, 245, exhibit 8.13.

10. From *Financial Management for Medical Groups*, 246, exhibit 8.14.

11. Adapted from *Financial Management for Medical Groups*, 249, exhibit 8.15.

12. From *Financial Management for Medical Groups*, 251, exhibit 8.16.

13. From *Financial Management for Medical Groups*, 252, exhibit 8.17.

14. From *Financial Management for Medical Groups*, 253, exhibit 8.18.

15. From *Financial Management for Medical Groups*, 254, exhibit 8.19.

16. From *Financial Management for Medical Groups*, 255, exhibit 8.20.

17. From *Financial Management for Medical Groups*, 257, exhibit 8.21.

Chapter 3

Accounts Payable, Accounting Systems, and Reconciliation

Payment of bills is popularly known as *accounts payable*, or A/P. Management of A/P requires knowledge of basic bookkeeping, accounting software, standard vendor payment processes, and internal cash controls in order to support an effective practice financial infrastructure.

Processing and Control of Accounts Payable

A/P are amounts owed to vendors and suppliers for goods and services acquired on a credit basis and for which the suppliers have not yet been paid. Usually these claims are unsecured and are frequently referred to as *open accounts*. The terms of these payable transactions normally require payment within 10 to 60 days after receipt of the goods or services.

Processing A/P includes maintaining a detailed record of individual accounts by vendor and using a system to identify dates on which the obligations should be paid. The terms of these transactions usually stipulate the taking of cash discounts, such as 2/10 net 30. (That is, if the invoice is paid within 10 days from the date of the invoice, the payer can take a 2 percent discount from the amount due; if the discount is not taken, then the total amount due is to be paid by 30 days from the date of the invoice.) Missing or not taking cash discounts can be costly, thus the system should ensure that all cash discounts are taken as offered.

A/P controls include ensuring that amounts due to vendors are authorized, authentic, and supported by underlying documentation, such as purchase orders and receiving reports, as well as invoices showing the complete details of the transaction. Before a payment is made on any account payable, the check signer should check the supporting evidence to ensure that unauthorized or erroneous disbursements are not being made.

Here are two hints for effective management of vendor accounts:

1. Ask suppliers to bill the medical group for all purchases on a set series of dates each month to prevent payments from bunching up and to ease the demands on cash outflows; and

2. Find out if vendors will grant a larger discount for paying cash at the time of purchase rather than being billed at a later date. Sometimes discounts up to 5 percent are possible.

Accounting Systems

An accounting system provides the basic structure for accumulating the practice's financial information. The amounts contained in financial statements and tax returns come from the accounting system. Historical information from the accounting system may be used to determine the amounts used in prospective statements, such as budgets and forecasts. Even if a practice uses zero-based budgeting and derives its budget from scratch, it still compares this budget against actual data from the accounting system.

The accounting system does not just provide information for financial reporting, it also supplies much of the information used for managerial decision making. For example, determining the break-even point or computing the cost of sending out a bill involves using data from the accounting system. The information used to compute physician bonuses or track expense accounts also comes from the accounting system.

An accounting system begins with a chart of accounts, which categorizes the various transactions that are recorded through payroll, A/P, the revenue cycle, and other sources. The transactions are then posted to the general ledger, which lists the activity for each account number in the chart of accounts and maintains the balance of cumulative activity for each account. The amounts from the general ledger provide the basis for the financial statements, tax returns, and many financial analyses.

Basic Financial Statements: An Overview

Before delving into the chart of accounts, it is important to understand the basic financial statements that your practice needs to create on a regular basis. These include the:

- Balance sheet;
- Income statement;
- Statement of changes in equity; and
- Statement of cash flows.

These financial statements may be prepared using the accrual basis of accounting in accordance with generally accepted accounting principles (GAAP) or some other comprehensive basis of accounting (OCBOA), such as the cash or tax basis. This chapter includes examples of both cash and accrual financial statements for Blue Mountain Orthopedic Group, P.C. (hereafter Blue Mountain),[1] a fictitious practice used only for illustration purposes (resemblance to any existing practice is purely coincidental).

Balance Sheet

The balance sheet tells what the practice owns (its assets), what it owes (its liabilities), and what its net worth or equity (its net claim on assets after subtracting liabilities) is. True to its name, the balance sheet must balance. The balance sheet equation is:

Assets = Liabilities + Equity

A *balance sheet* lists the assets and liabilities in the order of their liquidity (how quickly they convert to cash). The most liquid assets and liabilities are called *current assets and liabilities* because they are expected to convert to cash in less than one year. Examples of current assets include cash and A/R. Examples of current liabilities include A/P, payroll withholdings and accruals, and current maturities of long-term debt.

Blue Mountain's balance sheets (Exhibits 3.1 and 3.2) do not show any investments. If the practice had short-term investments, these would be included with the current assets. Any long-term investments would appear in a separate section between current assets and property and equipment.

A practice's long-term assets usually consist of medical equipment and other property such as computers, office furniture, and leasehold improvements. The balance sheet shows these items in a separate section, along with their cumulative depreciation and net book value.

Other long-term assets are those with an expected life greater than one year, other than investments, property, and equipment. These are included in the last group in the assets section. Examples include deposits and intangible assets such as goodwill.

Long-term liabilities appear in a separate section following the current liabilities. These include debts that the practice will pay in one year or more, such as long-term debt, net of current maturities. The equity section represents the owners' claim on net assets.

These amounts are the result of capital contributed by the owners, as well as the undistributed profits of the practice. The accounts in this section will vary depending on the type of entity. For example, corporate entities will show all classes of stock separately at par value beginning with common stock, followed by any contributed capital in excess of par, and retained earnings. Limited liability entities, partnerships, and sole proprietorships generally combine these amounts as members' capital, partners' capital, or proprietor's capital. Although one amount usually appears in these entities' balance sheets for capital, practices should keep detailed sub-accounts for each owner.

The retained earnings or owners' capital accounts should include the current-year net income, not just the undistributed amounts from prior years. This is true not only for the year-end financial statements, but also for interim statements. The related computation (adding current net income from the income statement to the equity account) is shown in the statement of changes in equity and posted to the balance sheet. This is the secret to balancing the balance sheet.

Exhibit 3.1
Accrual Basis Balance Sheet

Blue Mountain Orthopedic Group, P.C. Balance Sheet As of December 31, 2015 and 2014		
Assets		
Current assets:	**2015**	**2014**
Cash	$144,000	$86,000
Patient accounts receivable, net of allowance for doubtful accounts of $40,000 in 2015 and $35,000 in 2014	800,000	750,000
Prepaid expenses	35,000	25,000
Total current assets	979,000	861,000
Property and equipment, at cost:		
Leasehold improvements	50,000	50,000
Equipment	700,000	550,000
	750,000	600,000
Less: Accumulated Depreciation	285,000	210,000
Property and equipment, net	465,000	390,000
Other assets:		
Deposits	1,000	1,000
Total Assets	$1,445,000	$1,252,000

Exhibit 3.1
Accrual Basis Balance Sheet (continued)

Liabilities and Stockholders' Equity

Current Liabilities:

Current maturities of long-term debt	$40,000	$25,000
Accounts payable	38,000	35,000
Accrued payroll taxes	125,000	135,000
Accrued retirement plan contribution	115,000	110,000
Total current liabilities	318,000	305,000

Long-term Liabilities:

Long-term debt, less current maturities	135,000	85,000
Deferred taxes	326,000	283,000
Total long-term liabilities	461,000	368,000
Total Liabilities	779,000	673,000

Stockholders' equity:

Common stock, $1 par, authorized 20,000 shares:

issued and outstanding 7,000 shares	7,000	7,000
Contributed capital in excess of par	14,000	14,000
Retained earnings	645,000	558,000
Total stockholders' equity	666,000	579,000
Total Liabilities and Stockholders' equity	$1,445,000	$1,252,000

Exhibit 3.2

Income Tax Basis Balance Sheet for Cash Basis Taxpayer
Blue Mountain Orthopedic Group, P.C.

Statement of Assets, Liabilities, and Equities – Income Tax Basis
For the Years Ended December 31, 2015 and 2014

Assets	2015	2014
Current assets:		
Cash	$144,000	$86,000
Property and equipment, at cost:		
Leasehold improvements	50,000	50,000
Equipment	700,000	550,000
	750,000	600,000
Less: Accumulated Depreciation	435,000	290,000
Property and equipment, net	315,000	310,000
Other Assets:		
Deposits	1,000	1,000
	–	–
Total other assets	1,000	1,000
Total assets	$460,000	$397,000
Liabilities and Stockholders' Equity		
Current Liabilities:		
Current maturities of long-term debt	$40,000	$25,000
Accrued payroll taxes	125,000	135,000
Accrued retirement plan contribution	115,000	110,000
Total current liabilities	280,000	270,000
Long-term Liabilities:		
Long-term debt, less current maturities	135,000	85,000
Total Liabilities	415,000	355,000
Stockholders' equity:		
Common stock, $1 par, authorized 20,000 shares: issued and outstanding 7,000 shares	7,000	7,000
Contributed capital in excess of par	14,000	14,000
Retained earnings (deficit)	24,000	21,000
Total stockholders' equity	45,000	42,000
Total Liabilities and Stockholders' equity	$460,000	$397,000

Income Statement

Whereas the balance sheet shows the practice's assets, liabilities, and equity at a point in time, the income statement shows the entity's revenue, expenses, and net income over a period of time. The basic equation for the income statement is:

Revenues − Expenses = Net Income or (Loss)

The standard accounting period is one year. Any audit or review by an outside accounting firm would generally be performed on the annual financial statements. Ordinarily, a practice will also prepare interim financial statements on a monthly basis showing current month and year-to-date amounts on the income statement.

Operating revenues, such as fee-for-service income, capitation income, and other medical revenue, such as medical director fees, appear first on the income statement. GAAP requires that any significant amount of capitation revenue be shown separately from fee-for-service income.

The operating expenses appear next. These expenses relate directly to the production of operating revenues. Both GAAP and OCBOA allow an entity to organize, classify, and sub-classify these expenses in a useful or customary manner. One method that works well for most medical practices is to divide these expenses into staff salaries and fringe benefits, services and general expenses, purchased services, and provider-related expenses.[2] The presentation of physician salaries on a practice income statement varies. Corporate practices may include these with operating expenses or as a separate item (as is the case with Blue Mountain's financial statements). For partnerships, proprietorships, and limited liability entities, payments to physician-owners are generally considered "in kind" distributions of profit.

The income statement also includes income and expenses from sources other than operations: these include investment income, gains or losses on the sale of used medical equipment, and interest expense. Finally, after deducting income taxes, the income statement shows the practice's net income. Blue Mountain's income statement (Exhibit 3.4 and Exhibit 3.5) is combined with its statement of equity as in the next section.

Statement of Changes in Equity

The statement of changes in equity shows the activity in the capital accounts during the period and includes changes in both contributed capital and accumulated earnings accounts. Practices whose changes consist only of net earnings and distributions to owners often combine this statement with the income statement, as is the case with our Blue Mountain example (Exhibit 3.4 and Exhibit 3.5). Groups with more complex equity transactions, such as shareholder buy-ins or buyouts, generally report these transactions in a separate statement.

Statement of Cash Flows

The statement of cash flows explains the practice's sources and uses of cash during the year. The three categories are cash provided or used by:

1. Operating activities (the practice's normal business activities);

2. Investing activities (sales and purchases of investments, including equipment and other fixed assets); and

3. Financing activities (transactions involving the practice's debt and equity).

All of the entity's cash transactions fit into one of these three categories. The statement can present the section on operating activities using either the direct or indirect method. The direct method lists the gross amounts of the various operating cash receipts and disbursements. The indirect method starts with net income, then reconciles this number to cash flow from operations by adding or subtracting changes in the various current asset and liability accounts and noncash gains and losses, such as depreciation and gains or losses on the sale of fixed assets. Although the Financial Accounting Standards Board (FASB) recommends the direct approach, which is more intuitive, the indirect method (used in Exhibit 3.3) is typically easier for accountants to prepare and is more popular.[3]

Entities that use an OCBOA, such as the cash or tax method, are not required to prepare a statement of cash flows.

Exhibit 3.3
Statement of Cash Flows

Blue Mountain Orthopedic Group, P.C.
Statement of Cash Flows
As of December 31, 2015 and 2014

Cash Flows from Operating Activities:	2015	2014
Net Income	$87,000	$76,000
Depreciation	75,000	70,000
Deferred taxes	43,000	38,000
Changes in assets and liabilities:		
(Increase) decrease in accounts receivable	(50,000)	(80,000)
(Increase) decrease in prepaid expenses	(10,000)	2,000
Increase (decrease) in accounts payable	3,000	2,000
Increase (decrease) in payroll taxes payable	(10,000)	5,000
Increase (decrease) in retirement contributions payable	5,000	(10,000)
Net cash flows from operating activities	143,000	103,000
Cash Flows from Investing Activities:		
Purchase of leasehold improvements	–	(10,000)
Purchase of equipment	(150,000)	(25,000)
Net cash flows from investing activities	(150,000)	(35,000)
Cash Flows from Financing Activities:		
Repayment of short-term notes payable	–	(45,000)
Net Borrowings (repayment) of long-term debt	65,000	(25,000)
Proceeds from issuance of common stock	–	3,000
Net cash flows from financing activities	65,000	(67,000)

Exhibit 3.3 Statement of Cash Flows (continued)		
Increase (decrease) in Cash	58,000	1,000
Cash at Beginning of Year	86,000	85,000
Cash at End of Year	$144,000	$86,000

Bases of Accounting: Cash vs. Accrual

Medical practices generally use either the cash or the accrual method of accounting. The MGMA Cost Survey shows the annual percentage of practices using accrual method or cash method for tax purposes.[4] You can find the most recent report at the MGMA website (www.mgma.com).

The accrual method of accounting is consistent with GAAP. Its principles are determined primarily by the FASB, whose pronouncements constitute GAAP. Government-owned practices should also comply with pronouncements of the Governmental Accounting Standards Board. Other authoritative sources of GAAP include publications and pronouncements of the American Institute of Certified Public Accountants (AICPA). Finally, the usual accounting practices of a particular industry, such as the medical practice business, constitute GAAP for that industry, as long as they do not contradict official authoritative sources.

The AICPA's audit and accounting guide for the healthcare industry applies to all healthcare entities, including medical practices. This guide states that healthcare organizations should prepare their financial statements in accordance with GAAP.[5]

Despite that GAAP is the usual standard for financial reporting, the AICPA recognizes that for some businesses this method is too cumbersome. In certain situations, organizations may use other accounting methods. These other permissible accounting methods are known as OCBOA.[6]

Often practices prepare their financial statements on a basis that is consistent with the income tax regulations for cash basis taxpayers.

Accountants prefer calling these *tax basis* or *income tax basis* statements because the cash basis of accounting for income tax filing is better defined than the cash basis for financial reporting.

Both the cash and tax bases are considered OCBOA. Most physician-owned practices meet the criteria for issuing cash or tax basis financial statements.

Revenue and Expense Recognition: The Basic Difference

The basic and most important difference between the cash and accrual methods is the point at which each recognizes revenues and expenses. Accrual basis organizations recognize revenues when they are earned and expenses when they are incurred. Cash basis organizations recognize revenue when the cash is actually or constructively received and expenses when they are actually or constructively paid.

For a medical practice, this means that an accrual basis practice includes medical revenue on its income statement and the net value of any related A/R on its balance sheet at the time the physician sees the patient. A cash basis practice includes the revenue from the visit in its income statement when it receives payment for the services. It never shows the related A/R on its balance sheet.

Example 1

During March, Dr. Marcus sees a patient. The practice charges $110 for the services, and the patient pays a copayment of $20 at the time of service. The practice then bills the patient's insurance company, which has a negotiated allowed fee of $80 and the plan pays $60 in April. The related contractual write-off is $30.

An accrual basis practice would include $80 in revenue on the March income statement with a $60 net receivable on the March 31 balance sheet.

A cash basis practice would include $20 in revenue for March and $60 in revenue for April. The cash basis practice would never include the related A/R on its balance sheet.

An accrual basis practice would include the expenses related to the visit on the income statement during the period in which the service was performed. Any unpaid amount would be reflected as a liability on the practice's balance sheet until it is paid.

A cash basis practice would include the related expenses on its income statement during the period in which they are paid. A cash basis practice would not show the related liabilities, such as A/P or accrued payroll, on its balance sheet.

Example 2

During May, Suburban Family Practice, LLC, incurs $450 worth of laundry and linen expense. It pays this bill on June 10.

An accrual basis practice would include the $450 as an expense on its May income statement and as a liability (A/P) on its May 31 balance sheet.

A cash basis practice would include the $450 expense on its June income statement. It would never show this amount as a liability on its balance sheet.

Leaving A/R and A/P off their balance sheets does not relieve cash basis practices of the need to keep detailed accounting records for receivables and payables. They definitely should. Effective management of A/R and A/P is crucial for both accrual and cash basis practices. The difference is that cash basis practices don't include uncollected or unpaid amounts on their financial statements.

Refer to the sample financial statements in this chapter. Note that the accrual basis balance sheet (see Exhibit 3.1) includes A/R and A/P, whereas the tax/cash basis balance sheet (see Exhibit 3.2) does not. The differences in revenues and expenses between the two-income statements (Exhibits 3.4 and 3.5) reflect the timing differences between when these were earned or incurred and when the cash was received or paid. Exhibit 3.6 provides a reconciliation of the differences between the two sets of financial statements for the year 2015.

Cash Basis Exceptions for Recording Liabilities

Although cash basis practices do not generally accrue expenses, a couple of exceptions exist. First, tax laws allow all taxpayers, including cash basis taxpayers, to deduct qualified retirement plan contributions if they are made by the tax return due date (including extensions). Thus, the expense and liability for retirement plan contributions are generally the same whether the practice is cash or accrual based. Second, cash basis practices generally include unpaid payroll withholdings as liabilities on their balance sheets, and many accrue the employer's portion as well.

Depreciation

An accrual basis practice will make adjustments to its financial statements that are required by GAAP. A cash basis practice will usually make modifications to the strict cash basis of accounting that have substantial support, such as capitalizing fixed assets and recording the related depreciation. Tax basis depreciation expense may differ significantly from that reported on the accrual basis. This is because tax rules often allow accelerated depreciation write-offs in the early years of an asset's life, whereas GAAP generally requires a straight-line or a less aggressive accelerated method.

Deferred Taxes

While accrual basis practices must include GAAP depreciation on their financial statements, they often use accelerated methods for tax purposes. This creates a difference (potentially a significant one) between their financial statements and tax return net incomes. This is just one of many possible book-to-tax differences for accrual basis practices. GAAP requires that practices compute income taxes based on their GAAP income without regard to timing differences. The cumulative difference between the two income tax calculations appears on the balance sheet

Exhibit 3.4

Accrual Basis Statements of Income and Retained Earnings

Blue Mountain Orthopedic Group, P.C.
Statement of Income and Retained Earnings
For the Years Ended December 31, 2015 and 2014

	2015	2014
Revenues		
Net fee-for-service revenue	$6,930,000	$6,275,000
Capitation revenue	–	–
Other	55,000	50,000
Net revenue	6,985,000	6,325,000
Operating Expenses:		
Salary and Fringe Benefits:		
Staff salaries	1,200,000	1,100,000
Payroll taxes	100,000	90,000
Employee benefits	300,000	250,000
Total salary and fringe benefits	1,600,000	1,440,000
Services and General Expenses:		
Malpractice insurance	170,000	145,000
Provision for bad debts	180,000	175,000
Medical and surgical supplies	178,000	162,000
Depreciation	75,000	70,000
Rent	400,000	375,000
Information technology	100,000	95,000
Other general and administrative	388,000	367,000
Total services and general expense	1,491,000	1,389,000
Total operating expenses	3,091,000	2,829,000
Net revenue after operating expense	3,894,000	3,496,000
Provider-related expenses:		
Physician salaries and benefits	3,750,000	3,370,000
Net income after provider-related expenses	144,000	126,000
Other Income (Expense):		
Interest expense (net)	(12,000)	(8,000)
Net Income before income taxes	132,000	118,000
Provision for income taxes	45,000	42,000
Net income	87,000	76,000
Retained Earnings, Beginning of Year	558,000	482,000
Retained Earnings, End of Year	$645,000	$558,000

Exhibit 3.5

Income Tax Basis Statements of Income and Retained Earnings for a Cash Basis Taxpayer

Blue Mountain Orthopedic Group, P.C.
Statement of Revenues, Expenses, and Retained Earnings – Income Tax Basis
For the Years Ended December 31, 2015 and 2014

	2015	2014
Revenues:		
Net fee-for-service revenue	$6,700,000	$6,000,000
Capitation revenue		
Other	55,000	50,000
Net revenue	6,755,000	6,050,000
Operating Expenses:		
Salary and Fringe Benefits:		
Staff salaries	1,200,000	1,100,000
Payroll taxes	100,000	90,000
Employee benefits	300,000	250,000
Total salary and fringe benefits	1,600,000	1,440,000
Services and General Expenses:		
Malpractice insurance	180,000	150,000
Medical and surgical supplies	175,000	155,000
Depreciation	145,000	80,000
Rent	400,000	375,000
Information technology	100,000	95,000
Other general and administrative	388,000	367,000
Total services and general expense	1,388,000	1,222,000
Total operating expenses	2,988,000	2,662,000
Net revenue after operating expenses	3,767,000	3,388,000
Physician salaries and benefits	3,750,000	3,370,000
Net income after physician salaries and benefits	17,000	18,000
Other Income (Expense):		
Interest expense (net)	(12,000)	(8,000)
Net Income before income taxes	5,000	10,000
Provision for income taxes	2,000	4,000
Net income	3,000	6,000
Retained Earnings (deficit), Beginning of Year	21,000	15,000
Retained Earnings (deficit), End of Year	$24,000	$21,000

Exhibit 3.6
Cash-to-Accrual Adjustments 2015

Blue Mountain Orthopedic Group, P.C.
Cash-to-Accrual Adjustments
For the Year Ended 2015

Description	Cash		Debit		Credit	Accrual
			Adjustments			
Cash	144,000					144,000
Accounts receivable, net	0	A	800,000			800,000
Prepaid expenses	0	D	35,000			35,000
Leasehold improvements	50,000					50,000
Equipment	700,000					700,000
Accumulated depreciation	(435,000)	C	150,000			(285,000)
Deposits	1,000					1,000
						0
Notes payable						0
Current maturities of						
long-term debt	(40,000)					(40,000)
Accounts payable	0			B	38,000	(38,000)
Payroll taxes payable	(125,000)					(125,000)
Retirement contributions						
payable	(115,000)					(115,000)
Long-term debt, less						
current maturities	(135,000)					(135,000)
Deferred income taxes,						
long-term				F	326,000	(326,000)
Common stock	(7,000)					(7,000)
Contributed capital in						
excess of par	(14,000)					(14,000)
Beginning Retained Earnings	(21,000)	B	35,000	A	750,000	(558,000)
		F	283,000	C	80,000	
				D	25,000	
	3,000					87,000
Net fee-for-service revenue	(6,700,000)			A	50,000	(6,930,000)
				E	180,000	
Other	(55,000)					(55,000)
						0
Staff salaries	1,200,000					1,200,000
Payroll taxes	100,000					100,000
Employee benefits	300,000					300,000
Malpractice insurance	180,000			D	10,000	170,000
Provision for bad debts	0	E	180,000			180,000
Medical and surgical supplies	175,000	B	3,000			178,000
Depreciation	145,000			C	70,000	75,000
Rent	400,000					400,000
Information technology	100,000					100,000
Other general and						
administrative	388,000					388,000
Physician salaries and benefits	3,750,000					3,750,000
Interest expense	12,000					12,000
Provision for income taxes	2,000	F	43,000			45,000
						0
						0
						0
Net Income (Loss)	(3,000)					(87,000)
			1,529,000		1,529,000	

Exhibit 3.6
Cash-to-Accrual Adjustments 2015 *(continued)*

Explanation of Cash/Tax Basis to Accrual Adjustments

Item	Explanation
A	To add *net* accounts receivable to the balance sheet. Note that only the current-year change in this amount affects current-year income. The prior year amount is reflected in the beginning retained earnings difference.
B	To add accounts payable to the balance sheet. Note that only the current-year change in this amount affects current-year income. The prior year amount is reflected in the beginning retained earnings difference.
C	To adjust for difference in GAAP depreciation and the amount allowed for tax purposes. Note that only the current-year difference affects current-year income, while prior years' differences affect the beginning retained earnings, and the cumulative difference affects the accumulated depreciation amount.
D	To recognize the portion of unexpired malpractice insurance as an asset. Again, note that only the current-year difference affects the income statement, whereas the prior year difference affects beginning retained earnings.
E	To reclassify bad debt expense as an operating expense. For accrual basis financial statements, *net revenue* is net of contractual adjustments and charity care, but not net of bad debt expense. Because cash basis financial statements only report revenue when it is received (and bad debts are, by definition, never received), cash basis financial statements report net revenue net of contractual adjustments, charity care, *and* bad debts.
	This is a reclassification entry only; it does not affect the bottom line, except for timing differences in the real world.
F	To record the provision for deferred taxes. Again, note that only the current-year difference affects the income statement, whereas the prior year difference affects beginning retained earnings.

Examples of Other Differences Not Included in This Example

- Recognition of investment income;
- Capitalization, amortization, and impairment of intangible assets (i.e., goodwill);
- Accrued payroll, including vacation and sick pay;
- Accrual of claims payable and claims payable IBNR (incurred but not received); and
- Deferred revenue (revenue received in advance as a liability).

as deferred taxes. This amount may be an asset or a liability, depending on which tax expense is greater.

Other Differences

Many other differences between the bases of accounting exist. Because many cash basis practices report on the tax basis, some of these differences change when the related tax laws change.

Considerations in Selecting a Basis of Accounting

The Audit Myth

One pervasive myth holds that certified public accountants (CPAs) can only audit GAAP financial statements. This is not true. Statement on Auditing Standards No. 62 allows audits of OCBOA financial statements in certain situations and provides much of the authoritative guidance for reporting on the cash and tax basis.[7] The criteria in this standard would permit many medical practices to have audited cash or tax basis financial statements.

Revenue Determination

Net revenue is the largest item on most practice financial statements. Because of the differences between gross charges and the amount of revenue ultimately collected, the amount of net revenue on an accrual basis practice's income statement is an accounting estimate. The percentage of contractual write-offs and charity care can shift constantly because of changes in payer mix, fee schedules, deductibles, and economic conditions. The AICPA has cautioned that revenue amounts involving accounting estimates are a fraud risk and it has instructed auditors to exercise professional skepticism in auditing these amounts, particularly when they are tied to bonuses or other incentive compensation.[8] For example, a significant portion of the well-publicized fraud at HealthSouth was perpetrated by misstating contractual adjustments.[9] An accrual basis practice must devote the time and other resources necessary to ensure that these computations are reasonably accurate.

Taxes

Most physician-owned practices qualify to use the cash method for income tax purposes. This method usually saves or defers a significant amount of income taxes because the deferral of income tax on A/R is generally much larger than the deductions lost by not being able to deduct A/P and other accrued liabilities. Because Section 446(a) of the Internal Revenue Code requires that a taxpayer compute taxable income on the same basis of accounting it regularly uses in keeping its books,[10] these practices must also issue their external financial statements on the cash basis. Although a cash basis practice might prepare internal analyses that include accrual basis attributes for internal management purposes, it should ensure that the financial statements given to third parties, such as bankers, reflect the basis of accounting used in preparing its income tax returns.

Simplicity vs. Economic Reality

Many smaller practices and physician-owned practices that can use the cash method for tax purposes do so because it is easier than the accrual method. Conformity with GAAP involves more than merely adding A/R and A/P to the balance sheet. A practice could devote significant resources to computing deferred taxes, accrued vacation pay, the provision for bad debts, and other accrual items.

All these GAAP complexities not only increase the amount of time and other resources required to generate practice financial statements, but they often make the financial statements more difficult for individuals without a financial background, including many physician-owners, to understand.

Although cash basis financial statements may be easier for physician-owners to understand, they may not reflect economic reality. When accrual basis accounting records transactions are incurred, they result in matching revenues with the related expenses. Because the cash basis records these items when the cash changes hands, such matching is not guaranteed and the financial statements could be badly distorted, particularly for practices with more complex financial situations, such as capitation arrangements with operating liabilities for payments to other providers.

Chart of Accounts

Whether an organization is a public entity or a private business, it needs a set of statements to record its financial condition. The *chart of accounts*[11] is the starting point for every organization's financial records.

132

It lists the accounts that are used to record the organization's expenses and revenues as well as its assets and liabilities. The chart of accounts defines the level of detail that the organization's accounting system will record as information and also provides the vocabulary of the accounting system as it describes each account.

Accounting rules dictate the structure and content of the financial reports that describe an organization's current financial position to managers, owners and shareholders, creditors, and governmental bodies. Practice managers require accurate and consistent financial information for short-term and long-term strategic decision making while creditors need the same information to decide the level of lending risk, which determines the amount of the loan and interest rate that the organization is qualified to receive. Financial statements are also the basis for the tax return and other legal filings to local, state, and federal agencies.

To be useful to all the various users, accounting records need to be reliable, relevant, and consistent. *Reliable* means that the records are free from bias or error, faithfully represent the financial status of the organization, and are verifiable after the fact. Reliable also implies that financial records are neutral in their nature and can be replicated by different accountants using the same objective data and measurement techniques. Accounting records must also be relevant, meaning that the records have the information that decision makers need and are sufficiently prepared and distributed in a timely manner. These records should also reflect consistency, meaning that there is comparability across organizations and with previous time periods.

The chart of accounts lists each account with a corresponding number for the accounting system to track and define the detail for recording all financial transactions. Without a designated accounting code stated in the chart of accounts, it is impossible to track a revenue or expense item in the accounting records.

All business and public entities have legal requirements to maintain accurate and representative accounting records that accurately show the financial status of the organization. Likewise, all businesses and public entities need reliable, relevant, and consistent accounting information for managerial decision making. Healthcare organizations in particular have unique business requirements that dictate how financial information should be categorized. Medical groups need to understand their sources of revenue, how contractual discounts are applied, how expenses are incurred, and details of the costs incurred to provide services, which necessitates that medical groups use a chart of accounts developed to meet their specific needs.

Choosing the Proper Categories and Level of Detail

A chart of accounts designates an account for every revenue and expense item it needs to track. The specific accounts an organization needs in its chart of accounts depends somewhat on its size and organizational complexity. Generally, larger and more complex organizations need more accounts than smaller, less sophisticated entities. However, while additional accounts allow the practice to record its revenue and expense in greater detail, it is more costly to maintain a complex accounting system. In addition, if the accounting system records information in too much detail, the managerial uses of the information can be handicapped by the inability to easily interpret financial records.

The selection of the level of detail is an important aspect in the design of the organization's chart of accounts. A CPA will often suggest that a medical practice should use the generic chart of accounts that the CPA uses for other retail or service industry clients and not a chart of accounts designed specifically for medical groups. Although a generic chart of accounts can work for a medical practice, it is unlikely to meet its unique needs.

The MGMA chart of accounts is designed specifically to generate the financial reports that a medical practice requires for decision making, for lenders, and to meet governmental legal reporting and tax filing requirements. It also has the desired flexibility that allows practices to add or modify accounts without destroying the chart's ability to prepare financial statements and tax reports.

The MGMA chart of accounts is divided into five major sections:

1. Assets;

2. Liabilities;

3. Equity;

4. Revenues; and

5. Expenses.

These sections directly relate to the three major financial reports for communication and decision making: the balance sheet, the income statement, and the cash flow statement.

Each category has a block of numbers assigned to show the general classification of each financial account and is generally presented in a standard order, beginning with the accounts presented in the balance sheet (also called the *statement of financial position*) and then in the accounts that build the income statement for the organization, followed by the cash flow statement.

Balance Sheet: Assets

Assets are resources owned by the organization such as A/R, equipment, and property. Assets may be tangible, such as land, buildings, and equipment, or intangible, such as goodwill, patents owned by the organization, and licenses. The chart of accounts lists assets in descending order of liquidity. Cash and other assets that are easily converted to cash are listed first, fixed assets such as property and equipment are listed next, and intangible assets are listed last. Asset accounts in the MGMA chart of accounts start with the account number 1000 and are the first accounts listed.

Balance Sheet: Liabilities

Liabilities are debts or obligations owed by the practice to creditors, such as loans and A/P. These obligations come from the purchase of goods or services on credit or by obtaining a loan from a financial institution to finance the purchase of equipment or buildings. Current liabilities, the obligations that are due to be paid within one year, are generally listed first in the chart of accounts, with A/P, bank overdrafts payable, and payroll obligations (tax, insurance, retirement plan withholdings, and accrued payroll amounts) listed before other payables such as rent or insurance. Long-term liabilities such as construction loans, long-term notes, and capital leases follow current liabilities. Deferred revenue, deferred compensation, and severance plan obligations are listed last. Liability accounts in the MGMA chart of accounts start with account number 2000.

Balance Sheet: Equity Accounts

Equity accounts (sometimes called *fund balance* in nonprofit organizations) reflect the net financial worth of the organization and represent the residual value of an entity's assets after deducting its liabilities. In a for-profit business, the equity will be the ownership interest, and in a not-for-profit, it will represent the retained net asset value of the organization. Equity accounts in the MGMA chart of accounts start with account number 3000.

Income Statement: Revenue and Expenses

The accounts used to create the income statement accounts follow the statement of financial position accounts. The accounts used to describe operating revenue precede the expense accounts, and the final accounts reflect non-operating revenue, non-operating expenses, and income taxes. This sequence enables the chart of accounts to follow the same sequence as the income statement, with account numbers that start with 4000 reflecting revenue; operating expenses starting with 5000, 6000, 7000, or 8000; and non-operating revenue and expenses starting with 9000.

Revenues are inflows of cash and other items of value received by the practice. Different revenue accounts categorize income to the practice by source, whether it is from fee-for-service activity, the sale of medical material, capitation payment, or some other source. The revenue section of the MGMA chart of accounts also includes "adjustments and allowances" as a subcategory[16] because medical practices consider allowances and adjustments as offsets to revenue so they can understand the effect of the discounts required by government and insurance payers and to easily gauge the net revenue associated with operations.

Expenses reflect the resources consumed in the process of generating revenue for the practice. In the MGMA chart of accounts, operating expenses are the costs incurred in the process of providing medical services to the organization's patients. Operating expenses include support staff salaries and benefits, and the cost of temporary labor (accounts starting with 5000); general and administrative expenses (accounts beginning with 6000); clinical and ancillary services expenses (accounts beginning with 7000); physician and nonphysician provider expenses (accounts beginning with 8000); and non-medical revenue and expenses (accounts beginning with 9000).

Measuring Profitability

The design of the operating expense accounts allows for the quick and easy evaluation of practice profitability. In physician-owned medical groups, the compensation of the physician-owners is based on the amount that remains after all expenses are subtracted from total net revenue. By organizing the MGMA chart of accounts with physician compensation and benefits as the last series of accounts, the logical flow of financial information is maintained. This sequence also allows management to logically present the financial situation of the practice by simply sorting the practice's trial balance (a listing of all accounts) by the account number.

The Numbering System

In addition to a basic numbering system, a chart of accounts may contain additional digits indicating location, division, or other attributes. For example, a practice may include identifying digits to track the professional expenses of the individual physicians and key personnel.

The Basic Chart

The core digits in a chart of accounts are the ones that identify its basic description. "Furniture and fixtures" and "travel" are examples of

Exhibit 3.7

Basic Field — Financial Categories[12]

Account Number	Description
1000	Assets
2000	Liabilities
3000	Equity
4000	Operating Revenue
4500	Patient and Payer Refunds
5000	Operating Expenses – Support Staff
6000	General and Administrative Expenses
7000	Clinical and Ancillary Services
8000	Physician and Nonphysician Provider Expenses
9000	Nonmedical Revenue and Expenses and Provision for Conversion to Cash Basis Accounting

Exhibit 3.8

Statement of Financial Position (Balance Sheet) Account[13]

Account Number	Description
1000	Assets
1100–1500	Current Assets
1600	Investments – Long-Term
1700–1800	Noncurrent Tangible Assets
1900	Intangible and Other Noncurrent assets
2000	Liabilities
2100–2300	Current Liabilities
2400	Long-Term Liabilities
3000	Equity

descriptions that might identify the core section of the chart of accounts numbers.

The order of a chart of account's core digits generally follows the financial statement order, with the balance sheet accounts first and the income statement accounts second. Take a detailed look at the MGMA chart of accounts, which contains the basic account numbering system as shown in Exhibit 3.7.

The first digit in the basic field indicates the major financial statement category. The second digit more specifically classifies the account by indicating a subcategory within the major category. For example, Exhibit 3.8 shows the second digit classification of the balance sheet or statement of financial position accounts.

This chart of accounts uses the additional digits in the basic field to further refine the attributes of a particular account.

Additional Fields

A chart of accounts may also refine the definition of a particular account by adding additional fields to its basic chart. For example, a practice may add an additional field identifying the particular location and/or department connected with a specific account. A practice might also use a supplemental field to track expenditures relating to a specific physician. For example, a practice's account mask might look like this: XXXX.LL.PPP. In this example, "XXXX" represents the basic field, "LL" the location field, and "PPP" the physician identifier field. Assuming Dr. Green is physician "005," works at the East End Clinic (location "02"), and the basic account number for physician meetings is "8252," the cost of Dr. Green's meetings would be charged to account 8252.02.005.

A practice usually uses the "00" field for expenditures that it cannot attribute to a particular location, department, or physician.

Coding Structure

The numeric coding system used in the 6th edition of *MGMA Chart of Accounts* has four fields. Each field represents a different purpose of accumulating financial information and is designed to accommodate the varying degrees of financial sophistication present in medical groups. The chart of accounts starts with the four-digit basic field that provides the complete set of financial accounts and accommodates a limited degree of cost allocation and cost tracking. If a practice's financial information needs are not met with the basic field, three additional fields are available to accommodate the specific needs of the practice.

1. **Entity field:** allows a practice with multiple legal entities to "roll up" consolidated financial reports with great ease;

2. **Responsibility center field:** allows data to be accumulated by specific administrative cost centers, ancillary services centers, clinical departments, or locations; and

3. **Provider field:** accommodates collecting revenue or expense information for specific providers.

The four fields can be illustrated as follows:

Entity Field	Basic Field	Responsibility Center Field	Provider Field
00	0000	00	000

This design allows for any practice to use the same four-digit basic field with up to 99 different legal entities, 99 separate responsibility centers, and 999 providers.

Entity field. This two-digit field allows a practice with different legal entities to use the same chart of accounts and to simplify understanding its aggregate financial performance. For example, it is possible for a medical group to have a separate physician practice, ambulatory surgery center, imaging center, real estate entity, and research corporation. The use of the entity field allows each legal entity to have a separate financial statement, but the practice's managerial needs are met by a consolidated financial record of the aggregate organization. The entity field also simplifies the automation of accounting records, since each entity will have similar accounting information.

Basic field. This four-digit field is the core of the chart of accounts and is central to the financial data gathering process. It serves to describe the fundamental nature of the accounts (assets, liabilities, equity, revenues, and expenses) and allows the further recording of activity within each area. The design is a sequential ordering of accounts that follows the logical transactions of a medical group. The basic field meets the information objectives of general-purpose financial statements and tax returns and allows assessment of the financial status of the organization. The basic field accommodates the data collection for the MGMA Cost Survey and provides a limited degree of cost accounting.

Responsibility center field. This two-digit field is used to identify the responsibility centers that the practice wants to track as the source of revenue and/or expense. A practice may want to accumulate revenue or expense by internal department, location, or service to better manage the area and to improve decision making. The responsibility center field allows for direct tracking of costs and revenue for each specific area of the practice.

Provider field. This three-digit field is used much like the responsibility center field but for the purpose of direct tracing of revenue or expenses to an individual physician or nonphysician provider. Practices that use the provider field can accumulate expenses that relate directly to a provider (such as the personnel assigned to a doctor or the equipment and supplies used by a physician) and relate the direct costs to the revenue recorded for the provider.

Other Considerations in Setting Up a Chart of Accounts

The MGMA chart of accounts, designed specifically for healthcare organizations, is flexible enough that it can be used by a variety of practices. This chart of accounts is designed to facilitate completing MGMA Cost Surveys and benchmarking against MGMA survey data.

CPA firms often maintain a standard chart of accounts that they copy when creating a chart of accounts for a new client. Often these charts of accounts are flexible enough to be used throughout a wide variety of industries, including medical practices. Accounting firms might also have industry-specific standard charts of accounts. When working with a new client, it is easier for a CPA to use a standard chart of accounts than create a new one from scratch. If the CPA firm maintains the practice's general ledger and prepares its financial statements, the practice can save staff time at the firm (and hopefully lower accounting fees) by using the firm's standard chart of accounts. However, using a standard chart of accounts that is not specific to physician practices can result in a loss of valuable data, as well as an inability to compare the data to national benchmarks.

Accounting software vendors sometimes include sample charts of accounts with the purchase of software. Using the vendor's chart of accounts often makes setting up the accounting system easier and less time consuming.

Whether using a chart of accounts from MGMA, the practice's accounting firm, a software vendor, or one designed from scratch, the practice needs to devote sufficient time and resources to customizing this chart of accounts to meet its needs. A well-planned chart of accounts can facilitate better financial reporting, tax reporting, and management's ability to extract the data from the accounting system that it needs for decision making. A chart of accounts that is easy to set up or used by a variety of industries may be too basic to meet a practice's needs for extracting data from its system. A poorly designed chart of accounts can make the financial reporting and decision-making process unnecessarily cumbersome and time consuming for those who assemble the data. Conversely, a chart of accounts that is unnecessarily complex involves excessive time and resources to process accounting transactions. A tricky part of planning the chart of accounts is making it complex enough to provide good information for reporting and decision making, flexible enough to accommodate growth and change, and simple enough to eliminate unnecessary work for the accounting staff.

Recording Transactions: Journals, Modules, and Journal Entries

A practice engages in many financial transactions, which its accounting system should properly reflect. The accounting system needs to provide a mechanism for assigning the appropriate chart of accounts code to each of these transactions. Most transactions first enter the accounting system through what have historically been referred to as *journals* but are often referred to as *modules* in today's era of computerized accounting systems. Common journals or modules used by medical practices include payroll and A/P. Practices that carry significant quantities of medical supplies, drugs, or items for resale (i.e., glasses, lenses, or orthopedic devices) might also use an inventory module.

Accounting System Modules: Setup Considerations

When configuring an accounting system, practice personnel typically make decisions that control how transactions are classified. For example, when setting up payroll, the practice can generally specify the accounts to which certain payroll transactions post. Accounting systems often permit transactions to post in either detail or summary form. Posting in detail, the general ledger contains the details of the individual transactions. For example, the office-supplies account lists all of the individual invoices for office supplies rather than just the total of all invoices for the period. The advantage of summary posting is that the general ledger is smaller, and the disadvantage is that staff may need to go to the subsidiary records to obtain specific details. Some accounting systems have a *drilldown* feature that offers the best of both worlds; it is a condensed general ledger that provides details with the click of a mouse.

Understanding the Chart of Accounts Methodology Is Crucial

Because some of the decisions regarding chart of accounts coding are made on an ongoing basis, personnel who routinely use these modules should be familiar with the chart of accounts and its methodology. For example, although the A/P module frequently has a default chart of accounts code for each vendor, the appropriate account number often varies. A check written to a specific physician could be reimbursement for a meeting, entertainment expense, office supplies, or some other purpose. The addition of a new employee to the payroll module usually involves assigning an account for that employee's salary, for example, "salaries–billing" or "salaries–laboratory."

Even if a practice's outside accountant maintains the general ledger and prepares the financial statements, its administrator or other financial personnel usually need to be familiar with the chart of accounts. They are often responsible for communicating the proper chart of accounts codes for practice transactions to the accountant. Practice personnel also need to extract data from the ledger to perform financial analysis.

General Journal Entries: Recording Other Transactions

Although these modules or journals often produce the bulk of a practice's accounting transactions, the accounting system must have a mechanism for recording other financial transactions. The book or worksheets that contain entries of these transactions are referred to as the *general journal*.

A practice usually records depreciation on its fixed assets or its retirement plan accrual through a journal entry. It might also use a journal entry to correct the account number to which a particular transaction was charged. One way that a practice that outsources its payroll might record summary payroll information with a general journal entry.

Transferring Revenue Cycle Data to the Accounting System

Most practices use a practice management system to bill charges and manage A/R. Some practices have an interface between their practice management system and their accounting system, which allows billing activity to post automatically to the general ledger. Other practices record billing, collections, and other A/R information through a journal entry. The billing system can usually produce a report that summarizes the information necessary to make the journal entry. The nature in which the practice records this data varies significantly depending on whether the practice is a cash basis or accrual basis practice.

General Ledger

The general ledger lists activities for each account in the chart of accounts. This information comes from other journals or modules, such as the payroll, A/P, or the general journal. The process of transferring or entering this activity in the general ledger is referred to as *posting*. In addition to containing a list of activities, each account has a *balance* at any given point in time. All transactions either increase or decrease this balance. Accounting systems use *debits* and *credits* to signify whether a particular transaction increases or decreases an account's balance. A debit increases the balance of an asset or expense account, whereas a credit decreases the balance of these accounts. Conversely, credits increase liability, equity, and revenue accounts, whereas debits decrease these accounts.

Asset and expense accounts normally have a debit balance, whereas liability, equity, and income accounts normally have a credit balance. This is referred to as the account's *normal* balance. When reviewing the general ledger, the administrator and other practice personnel should be alert for accounts that do not have a normal balance. For example, a credit balance in cash indicates an overdraft. A debit balance in a liability account indicates a potential overpayment. Balances that are not *normal* may indicate accounting errors that need to be corrected.

Exhibit 3.9 shows, for the major financial statement classifications, whether a debit or credit increases or decreases the account and the normal account balance.

Finally, for every accounting transaction, the debits should equal the credits. Consequently, the sum of the account balances should equal zero. When the general ledger totals do not equal zero, it is out of balance, and the financial statements will also be out of balance. Accounting personnel will need to find the error and make appropriate corrections.

Exhibit 3.9

The Effect of Debits and Credits on Major Financial Statement Classifications

Financial Statement Classification	Increase	Decrease	Normal Balance
Asset	Debit	Credit	Debit
Liability	Credit	Debit	Credit
Equity	Credit	Debit	Credit
Income	Credit	Debit	Credit
Expense	Debit	Credit	Debit

Financial Statement Preparation

The amounts on a practice's balance sheet and its income statement come directly from its general ledger. Often, the balances of similar accounts are combined to create one line item on the financial statements. For example, a practice may have several cash accounts, but only one amount for cash on its balance sheet. To prepare the statement of cash flows, accounting personnel must go beyond the general ledger and analyze cash flow and/or other account activity. Preparing the statement of changes in equity may also involve additional analysis.

The Closing Process

At the end of the accounting year, practice personnel should expand on normal month-end procedures to ensure that ending balances are correct. For example, while a practice may record an estimated provision for depreciation on a monthly basis, it should ensure that the final depreciation balance matches the amount on its updated depreciation schedule. If the practice has an outside accountant report on the year-end financial statements, it will need to post any adjustments the accountant may have to the general ledger.

To close its books for the year, a practice must adjust all income statement accounts to zero and transfer the balance of these accounts (which is the practice's profit or loss for the year) to an equity account.

(For a corporation, this account is retained earnings.) Most computerized systems perform this function automatically when selecting a year-end closing option, although the practice may need to stipulate the specific equity account(s) to which the transfer should be made.

After completing the closing process, the practice is ready to record transactions for the next year. All income statement accounts begin the year with a zero balance, while the ending balance sheet amounts for the old year will be the beginning balances for the new accounting year. This is because the balance sheet reflects amounts at a point in time, whereas the income statement reports the totals for a period in time.

Reconciliations

Reconciliations compare actual quantities against control records. For example, the practice might compare the actual quantity of medical supplies on hand against perpetual inventory records and investigate any differences. A group might compare the number of procedures billed for a service to the number of supply units expensed for that specific procedure. Cash drawers should be reconciled at least daily.

A *bank reconciliation* compares the balance per the bank with the balance per the accounting records and accounts for all differences, such as outstanding checks. A practice's cash account or bank account is one of the areas most susceptible to fraud. Because of the risk associated with bank accounts, it is imperative to perform timely bank reconciliations so that any banking irregularities can be detected quickly. Bank reconciliations have traditionally been done monthly, but the fact that this information is available online allows a practice to balance its bank account at almost any point in time. Because of today's large amounts of electronic deposits and debits, many practices need to reconcile this balance frequently. For example, practices may need to compare the amount actually deposited in the bank against a payer's electronic remittance information.

Segregation of Duties

By dividing the duties associated with a particular area among different people, a practice reduces the risk of inappropriate activities. This typically involves separating the responsibilities for authorizing a transaction, recording the transaction, and physically handling the related asset. For example, the employee who orders supplies should not open the mail (which contains the related invoices), pay bills, receive the supplies, or maintain custody of the key to the supply cabinet. The employee who opens the mail and makes the bank deposit should not post payments or enter adjustments to patient accounts.

Although a small practice with limited business office staff may have difficulty accomplishing sufficient segregation of duties, this is usually possible. Using a bank lockbox and receiving payments electronically can improve control over cash receipts by preventing staff members who record the related transactions from physically accessing the payments.

Having physician-owners or outside accountants perform some of the incompatible functions may accomplish sufficient segregation of duties. For example, assigning a physician-owner or outside accountant to receive an unopened bank statement and review it before giving it to accounting personnel provides a check over A/P and bank account activity. When the practice administrator or another employee with other responsibilities for deposits or checks performs the bank reconciliations, it is critical that someone else reviews them.

Practice administrators sometimes serve as authorized check signers for their practices. Although this works well in some practices, it may create poor segregation of duties if the administrator performs incompatible A/P or checking account functions. A dishonest administrator who signs checks and handles A/P record-keeping can misappropriate funds, particularly when this administrator also reconciles the bank account. Requiring dual signatures on all checks or on checks in excess of a certain minimum amount can also improve control over disbursements.

Although using a facsimile signature stamp may expedite check processing, it can also reduce the effectiveness of internal control because anyone who has access to the facsimile signature stamp has the ability to approve a transaction. If the employee who prepares A/P checks has access to the facsimile signature stamp, this person has the ability to authorize, account for, and physically handle cash disbursements.

A practice should seriously consider whether using a facsimile signature poses an internal control risk. The stamp should be locked up with access given only to those with the authority to approve cash disbursements and who have no incompatible cash or A/P responsibilities. A more detailed discussion about segregation of duties is provided in Chapter 6 of this volume.

Conclusion

Management of A/P is an ongoing requirement for practice success. The key knowledge and skills necessary to manage this function include a basic understanding of bookkeeping, internal cash controls, and vendor payment models as well as skill in negotiating payment terms, reconciling accounts, and supervising A/P processes.

Notes

1. These sample financial statements were adapted from the online course materials for *Financial Management Boot Camp: Self-Study* (Englewood, CO: Medical Group Management Association, 2014), www.mgma.com/store/education/online/courses-self-study/ financial-management-boot-camp-self-study.

2. D. Gans, S. Andes, and R. Gold, *MGMA Chart of Accounts*, 6th ed. (Englewood, CO: Medical Group Management Association, 2014).

3. Thomas P. Edmonds, Frances M. McNair, Edward E. Milam, and Philip R. Olds, *Fundamental Financial Accounting Concepts* (New York: McGraw-Hill, 2003), 582–583.

4. *MGMA Cost Survey: 2014 Report Based on 2013 Data* (Englewood, CO: MGMA, 2014).

5. American Institute of Certified Public Accountants, *AICPA Audit and Accounting Guide: Health Care Organization* (New York: American Institute of Certified Public Accountants, 2006).

6. M. Ramos, *Preparing and Reporting on Cash and Tax Basis Financial Statements* (New York: American Institute of Certified Public Accountants, 1998), 3.

7. Ramos, *Preparing and Reporting*, 3–11.

8. American Institute of Certified Public Accountants, *Audit Risk Alerts: Health Care Industry Developments: 2003/04* (New York: American Institute of Certified Public Accountants, 2003), 76.

9. Michael Wynne, "HealthSouth: Overview and Entry Web Page," last modified June 2009, www.bmartin.cc/dissent/documents/health/access_healthsouth.html.

10. "Electronic Code of Federal Regulations," U.S. Government Publishing Office, March 23, 2015, www.ecfr.gov/cgi-bin/text-idx?rgn=div8&node=26:6.0.1.1.1.0.4.13.

11. Most of this "Chart of Accounts" section (and its subsections) is from Gans et al., *MGMA Chart of Accounts*, with some modifications.

12. Gans et al., *MGMA Chart of Accounts.*

13. Gans et al., *MGMA Chart of Accounts.*

Chapter 4

Managing Payroll

Aside from physician salaries, a practice's largest expense item is usually staff salaries, associated payroll taxes, and employee benefits. Most financial managers may not get involved intimately with the preparation of the payroll or the payroll tax returns. Rather, many groups rely on an outside payroll service organization to write payroll checks, to keep detailed employee records related to payroll data, to file federal and state tax returns, and to provide employees with relevant documentation as needed. In cases where an outside service is used, the financial manager should have a general knowledge about payroll matters so that the service can be properly supervised. Also, the financial manager should be able to answer questions from staff members about payroll without contacting the outside service.

Key skills for payroll management include establishing policies and procedures, overseeing the reporting system to capture work hours, comparing benchmarks, reporting taxes, and establishing guidelines for the payroll deduction process. Although many practices employ external organizations to implement payroll processing and reporting, it is essential for any practice manager to understand the overall flow, regulatory requirements, and functions of a high-performing payroll system.

The payroll process has three main steps:

1. Paying the employee;

2. Paying the employer portion of payroll taxes and transferring employee-deducted taxes to relevant government authorities; and

3. Filing tax reporting forms with relevant government authorities.

Some of the related payroll areas that financial managers should gain familiarity with include:

- Federal wage and hour requirements, including:
  - Exempt and nonexempt employees;
  - Minimum wage requirements;
  - Overtime pay;
  - Employer records;
  - Workers with disabilities;
  - Termination; and
  - Leaves of absence.
- Discrimination, including:
  - Federal legislation (e.g., Civil Rights Act) regarding prohibited actions, sexual harassment, and employer obligations;
  - Age discrimination;
  - Disabilities;
  - Affirmative action; and
  - National Labor Relations Board provisions about prohibited practices and penalties.
- Payroll requirements, including:
  - Federal and state income tax;
  - Federal Insurance Contributions Act (FICA) tax;
  - Deposit of payroll taxes;
  - Federal (FUTA) and state (SUTA) unemployment taxes;
  - Federal and state tax returns; and

- – Workers' compensation regulations and requirements.
- Employee deferrals and deductions relating to benefits, such as:
  - – Health insurance;
  - – 401(k) plans;
  - – Short and long-term disability insurance; and
  - – Flexible and dependent spending accounts.
- Post-employment issues, including:
  - – Consolidated Omnibus Budget Reconciliation Act of 1985 (COBRA) qualifications and payments.

Payroll administration includes managing employee personnel and payroll information, including accruals, and compliance with federal, state, and local employment laws.

Financial managers should obtain copies of relevant payroll-related laws and regulations and may want to subscribe to a payroll information service to gain access to an ongoing stream of updated information. If an outside service is used, this information should be provided to the practice by the servicing firm.

Payroll Methods

The process of payroll can occur using one of three methods:

1. The practice prepares the employees' payroll internally;
2. The practice hires a certified public accountant (CPA) and/or bookkeeper to process the payroll checks; or
3. The practice outsources payroll to a payroll vendor.

According to the government, the employer is ultimately responsible for ensuring that payroll has been processed accurately and that taxes have been filed appropriately. Therefore, it is imperative that you have a good working knowledge of payroll and the tax laws. Payroll reports should be reviewed at least each payroll cycle.

Processing payroll internally usually requires the purchase of software with this capability. Many smaller practices use this option, although it can be risky if the practice does not have a staff member who is or has become proficient in payroll requirements.

If you hire a CPA or bookkeeper to process payroll, you must ensure that the person performing the duties is, in fact, experienced and knowledgeable.

Outsourcing payroll has become more popular in the past few years as the tax laws have become more complicated. Payroll firms have already developed policies and procedures surrounding the process and, presumably, should be current on any changes in the tax laws. In addition, they may be more sophisticated with reporting. However, outsourcing firms may not be able to readily provide you with data in the format that you request, unless it offers a flexible design. For instance, each type of paid hour such as regular, overtime and time off, i.e., jury duty, vacation and bereavement, should have a unique designation for input and reporting. It may also be more difficult to communicate your needs easily with a large firm.

Tax Considerations

Payroll is a type of accounts payable. The employer pays employees' wages after withholding the employees' portion of payroll taxes. The employer then calculates its own portion of payroll taxes and transfers employee and employer taxes to appropriate taxing authorities. Solo physicians or small groups may do their own payroll, but then they are also responsible for payroll taxes, and that could be a hassle. These days, a number of banks offer payroll services at a nominal cost. This takes a lot of responsibility away from smaller groups. Some tax considerations include:

- **Federal withholding taxes.** These are determined from the required W-4 form completed by all new employees.

- **Social Security.** It is also known as FICA or OASDI, which stands for Old-Age, Survivors, and Disability

Insurance. The current employee tax rate can be found on the Social Security website. The employer is required to match the employee's contribution.

- **Medicare.** As of 2013, both the employee and the employer are taxed at a rate of 1.45 percent each. The Patient Protection and Affordable Care Act established a new Additional Medicare Tax of 0.9 percent that also went into effect in 2013. The new *Additional Medicare Tax* applies to single individuals earning more than $200,000 and married couples filing jointly who earn more than $250,000. However, employers must withhold the Additional Medicare Tax from all workers, regardless of marital status, on wages exceeding $200,000. Thus the employee Medicare tax rate, normally 1.45 percent, will rise to 2.35 percent on earnings higher than $200,000 regardless of the filing status. The employer Medicare tax rate remains 1.45 percent.[1] There is no taxable wage limit for Medicare taxes. Remember to always check with your CPA or tax professional or the government website for the most up-to-date tax rates.

- **State withholding taxes.** The percentage varies by state and several states do not have withholding taxes. Check with your state for your withholding requirements. As of this writing, states with no state income tax are:
  - Alaska;
  - Florida;
  - Nevada;
  - New Hampshire;
  - South Dakota;
  - Tennessee;
  - Texas;
  - Washington; and
  - Wyoming.

- **Federal Unemployment Tax Act.** This tax is paid on the first $7,000 in wages per employee and may be as low as 0.8 percent depending on the timeliness of submission.[2]

- **State Unemployment Insurance.** This varies depending on the employer's experience rating. Usually, this is paid by the employer, but some states require the employees to contribute to this tax as well.

- **Local taxes.** These vary depending on requirements of the jurisdiction, city, or county.

Tax laws and regulations change frequently and vary widely based on number of staff members, geographic location, exempt status, and regulations. Whether you calculate your payroll in house or contract with an outside accountant or payroll service, it is the employer's responsibility to report and pay taxes based on the federal and state laws. Timeliness and accuracy are critical. Vendors and software will help you calculate accurately, but you have to make sure that deposits are made on time. Inaccurate or late deposits can result in penalties and interest charges. Employers who fail to comply with these requirements may be subject to civil and/or criminal tax penalties.

Most states require state income taxes to be withheld on earnings. To be compliant, you must check with your state for the exact withholding requirements.

Some local entities (city, county, or school districts) also have withholding and reporting requirements. Like the states, most local entities have patterned their laws after federal tax codes.

Taxes must be paid and filed to the appropriate federal and state agencies according to very specific schedules, depending on the tax liability. It is critical for you to determine when and where you need to file in order to avoid penalties.

In general, a practice will need to report the payroll taxes on a quarterly basis on Form 941 (Employer's Quarterly Federal Tax Return). After you file your first Form 941, you must file a return for each quarter even if you have no taxes to report, until a final return is filed as explained in the Instructions to Form 941.

At year end, W-2 forms (Wage and Tax Statements) need to be sent or delivered to each employee, with copies filed with the Social Security Administration and copies held by the employer.

State unemployment taxes generally must be filed on a quarterly basis. While federal unemployment tax returns are filed annually, the taxes will probably need to be deposited quarterly. In the event of noncompliance with the timely filing of payroll taxes, the assessed penalties can be extreme. Most payroll services indemnify the client if taxes are transmitted late or incorrectly calculated.

Another type of penalty is the *trust fund recovery penalty*. These penalties can be assessed against individuals who are responsible for obtaining and paying the taxes (e.g., accountants, owners, administrators, etc.).

Penalties are nondeductible, so the practice is basically paying taxes on its taxes. A delay in paying taxes should never be considered in financial management.

Internal Revenue Code

Practices must comply with employment tax rules and procedures contained in the Internal Revenue Code. The following issues must be considered:

- Determining whether the federal tax coverage rules apply;
- Computing an employee's taxable wages;
- Calculating the employment taxes to be withheld and paid by the employer;
- Depositing the correct amount of employment taxes with the government; and
- Filing tax returns.

Policies and Procedures

A practice must decide on these criteria to process payroll:

- Exempt and nonexempt status of each staff member;
- Pay rates or scales for each of the practice's job classifications;
- Policies for breaks, lunches, time off, and how pay is to be addressed;
- Payroll cycle and frequency (typically every two weeks, but this may vary);
- What day staff members are paid and how checks are distributed;
- Availability and requirements for direct deposit;
- Payroll deductions for employee insurance plans, such as health, dental, vision, life, accident and illness, and disability;
- Retirement plan, 401(b), or 403(b) contributions;
- Donations or contributions to community organizations (e.g., United Way);
- Mandated deductions such as garnishments, child support, or tax levies; and
- Payment of any overtime or shift differentials.

Payroll Reporting System

The practice should have a formal process by which staff members can report hours worked and/or hours off for each pay period. Typically the pay period will be recorded in two-week increments with 40 hours per week.

Generally a practice will keep a time clock near the employee entrance that allows for a paper time card to be punched or the information can be entered electronically or digitally into the payroll system. Biometric time clocks, such as those that require an employee's fingerprint, can be used to prevent the buddy punch, in which employees "clock in" for other employees.

The payroll reporting system should:

- Record time off for vacations, sick leave, meetings, jury duty, and/or bereavement;
- Reflect the practice's policies and procedures relating the matrix of different types of paid time off, time accrued in each category as well as the past cycle's hours utilized and paid;
- Create reports for tracking and identifying hours worked and time off by each individual;
- Calculate and report pension deferrals and benefits contributions and report the remaining taxable income accurately;
- Calculate and report taxes paid by the practice;
- Calculate and report taxes withheld from the employee; and
- Generate end-of-year tax documents for employees and the practice.

Conclusion

Effective management of payroll systems is a significant part of the infrastructure that supports the entire clinical enterprise. Obviously, employees expect to be paid regularly and without bureaucratic hurdles. In addition, external taxing agencies and certain regulators have a stake in the timely payment of payroll and associated record-keeping systems. The effective administrator employs knowledge of federal regulatory requirements, as well as the ability to establish effective payroll policies and reporting routines.

Notes

1. "The New 0.9% Medicare Surtax and 3.8% Tax on Net Investment," Cherry Bekaert LLP, 2014, www.cbh.com/guide/the-new-0-9-medicare-surtax-and-3-8-tax-on-net-investment/.

2. "Topic 759: Form 940: Employer's Annual Federal Unemployment (FUTA) Tax Return: Filing and Deposit Requirements," U.S. Internal Revenue Service (IRS), last modified March 6, 2015, www.irs.gov/taxtopics/tc759.html.

Chapter 5

Creating and Managing Budgets

Budgeting Basics

Budgeting is an accounting and planning tool that practices use to plan for the future. Key skills required to effectively manage budgets include understanding of basic accounting principles and budgeting methodologies, as well as forecasting capital needs, conducting financial analyses, benchmarking, and communicating financial results to key stakeholders. By taking the time to prepare a budget, a practice can anticipate potential problems, such as cash shortages, and prepare for them. Practice leaders can identify potential opportunities and plan to capitalize on them. A budget provides a framework for monitoring and evaluating operational and accounting performance. Approved budgets improve organizational efficiency by authorizing expenditures of practice resources, thus avoiding multiple requests for approval of these items. Finally, an effective budget process facilitates communication within the practice because it involves key people in different departments and functions across the operation.

Budgeting vs. Financial Accounting

Although budgets depend on financial accounting systems, they are different in some important ways. While the accounting system reports transactions that happened in the past, a budget anticipates transactions

163

that will happen in the future. Financial statements focus on external reporting and must be presented in a format prescribed by generally accepted accounting principles (GAAP) or some other comprehensive basis of accounting (-), such as the cash or tax basis. Conversely, due to the fact that budgets focus on the internal needs of management, administrators may tailor the format of budgets to fit the needs of the organization.

The Budget's Relationship to Strategic and Operational Planning

Strategic planning is the development of a long-range course of action (i.e., 5 to 10 years) to achieve the medical group's goals. Operational planning is the development of short-term plans to achieve goals identified in the strategic plan. Operational plans cover periods ranging from one week or a month to several years. Budgeting is the financial portion of the operational plan as it defines the resources available to attain the practice's short-term and long-term goals.

To benefit from the budget process, a practice should first have a strategic plan and establish its goals for the budget period. In some cases, the administrator may need to begin the budget process as a basis for stimulating discussion to assist the board in establishing its objectives.

The Budget Process

Many people consider budgets to be an activity that an administrator or finance department carries out in isolation, without consulting the rest of the practice; this assumption is far from true. Although the administrator or a key financial representative usually has overall responsibility for preparing and coordinating the budget, the process is most beneficial when key clinical and administrative personnel, physicians, and other members of the governing body engage in the process and refer to the organization's operational and strategic plans.

In smaller practices, the outside accountant may occasionally assist in this process, but in most cases, the role of an outside accountant in the budget process should be purely that of an advisor or facilitator as those key stakeholders within the organization insiders should determine the organization's objectives and control its related budget process.

Obtain Data from Department Managers

The administrator (or other designated budget coordinator) reviews the practice's goals and objectives, determines what data are needed, and prepares the working documents necessary for obtaining this information. As a general rule, the administrator should delegate the task of gathering budget amounts to the lowest level appropriate, such as department managers for the cost and expense budgets and the patient accounting manager for revenue amounts. Due to the sensitive and confidential nature of physician compensation, the administrator or a key financial person normally prepares the provider compensation budget.

Assemble Budget and Revise as Necessary

After receiving requested data from key clinical and administrative personnel, the administrator assimilates it into budget form or template. The administrator identifies problem areas and inconsistencies with the numbers as compared to the practice's goals and modifies the budget in coordination with the participants and governing body. Business plan revisions may be necessary if desired physician compensation or other objectives are incompatible with financial realities.

Board Approval

After assembling a budget that is consistent with the organization's goals and financial realities, the administrator presents it to the governing body for approval. During this approval process, the administrator should be adequately prepared to describe the budget development process that occurred, explain any significant changes especially market changes that may impact the previous year's or actual results, and make any updates or revisions after board input.

Ongoing Monitoring and Revisions

Throughout the budget period, the practice monitors the actual results vs. the budget projections and stays alert for changes in the operating environment that necessitate changes to the budget or operations, developing action plans with specific timelines and tactics needed to address any variances.

To assist practice leadership in monitoring the budget, many accounting systems have report-writing features, such as a comparison of income statement balances against the budget. Many client accounting software packages enable users to produce these types of statements, so practices that use an outside accountant to prepare financial statements can most likely request and receive these reports.

Types of Budgets

Although the term *budget* implies a single process, a practice often needs several budgets to address its specific needs. The practice's mission, structure, and approach to management determine the different types of budgets it needs to fulfill its strategic and operational plans. Several of the exhibits contained in this chapter show the various budgets used by a hypothetical practice, Deep South Obstetrics and Gynecology, P.C. This practice is purely fictitious; any resemblance to an existing practice is a coincidence.[1]

Revenue Budget (May Incorporate Separate Statistics Budget)

The revenue budget is the usual starting point for the budget process. Many of the amounts determined in other parts of the budget process depend on the revenue budget. Some practices prepare a separate statistics budget that forecasts provider production levels, while other practices incorporate this process into their revenue budget.

The revenue budget combines volume information from the statistics budget with projected reimbursement information. Practice personnel need to exercise care in determining revenue budget amounts. Changes in payer fee schedules, payer mix, CPT coding rules, deductibles, changes in RVU valuation and the practice's chargemaster can change the dollar amount of reimbursement, as well as the gross collection rate often used to compute budget revenues. Additional considerations are projected capitation income, ancillary revenue, and other income sources (e.g. investments).

Note that the revenue budget in Exhibit 5.1 takes into consideration overall volume growth, as well as volume generated by a new physician and other revenue. This sample budget revises the expected gross collection rate of the practice based on the anticipated collection rates and payer mix. In addition to the amount of revenue available to the practice, the revenue budget needs to forecast when the revenue will be received. Depending on the nature of a practice, its basis of accounting (cash or accrual), and its budgets, either the master budget or the cash budget will need to include these amounts.

Statistics Budget

The advantage of having a separate statistics budget is that it provides uniform assumptions regarding volume of services, types of services, rate of inflation, and so forth, for all of the practice's budgets.

Accurate volume estimates are critical to the success of the entire budget process for a medical practice. Unfortunately, predicting volume is often difficult because the number and type of patients depend on many factors, some within the control of the practice and some outside of its control. Marketing campaigns, new managed care contracts, termination of managed care contracts, seasonality, area business expansion, and demographic shifts in the community are only some of the activities that can affect practice volumes. It is imperative that you are aware of any potential retirement, reduction in FTE status and other changes in the production of your current providers. If it overestimates volume, a practice might increase overhead expenses and therefore reduce the practice's net income. If a practice underestimates volume, it risks losing patients to competitors and incurring increased operating costs caused by staff overtime and inefficiencies resulting from overcrowding.

Capital Budget

The capital budget is used to plan for purchases of assets that have useful lives greater than one year. For example, a cardiology practice

Exhibit 5.1
Revenue Budget

DEEP SOUTH OBSTETRICS AND GYNECOLOGY, P.C.
Revenue Budget

Description/Month		Jan	Feb	Mar	Apr	May	Jun
Charges 2013		820,000	685,000	855,000	825,000	845,000	805,000
2014 growth	3%	24,600	20,550	25,650	24,750	25,350	24,150
New doctor							
Charges 2014		844,600	705,550	880,650	849,750	870,350	829,150
Projected collections rate							
−2013 charges 51.7%							
−2014 charges 52.5%							
Collections 2014		409,981	417,285	417,785	402,512	456,576	449,818

Payer	Collection Rate	Mix	Weighted Collection Rate
Medicare FFS	52%	23%	11.96%
Medicare HMO	47%	5%	2.35%
Commercial HMO	53%	34%	18.02%
Commercial PPO	57%	25%	14.25%
Commercial	60%	4%	2.40%
Medicaid	40%	6%	2.40%
Self-pay	37%	3%	1.11%
		100%	52.49%

Other Revenue
Contract Ultrasounds

	Jan	Feb	Mar	Apr	May	Jun
Studies per Month	100	90	105	95	105	100
Rate	200	200	200	200	200	200
Revenue	20,000	18,000	21,000	19,000	21,000	20,000
Other Revenue	3,750	3,750	3,750	3,750	3,750	3,750
Total Other Revenue	23,750	21,750	24,750	22,750	24,750	23,750

Jul	Aug	Sep	Oct	Nov	Dec	Total
755,000	780,000	810,000	860,000	800,000	780,000	9,620,000
22,650	23,400	24,300	25,800	24,000	23,400	288,600
	25,000	40,000	60,000	70,000	60,000	255,000
777,650	828,400	874,300	945,800	894,000	863,400	10,163,600
449,278	425,760	417,512	443,260	472,056	486,934	5,248,756

95	95	105	105	100	90	1,185
200	200	200	200	200	200	
19,000	19,000	21,000	21,000	20,000	18,000	237,000
3,750	3,750	3,750	3,750	3,750	3,750	45,000
22,750	22,750	24,750	24,750	23,750	21,750	282,000

Exhibit 5.2
Capital Budget

DEEP SOUTH OBSTETRICS AND GYNECOLOGY, P.C.

Capital Budget — 2014

Loc.	Description	Vendor	Computers	Off. Equip.
	Excess buildout			
	Satellite office furniture			
	Waiting	Office Inc		
	Nurses/MA station	Office Inc		
	Front desk	Office Inc		
	Medical records	Office Inc		
	Ultrasound room	Office Inc		
	Exam rooms (3)	PSS		
	Dictation room	Office Inc		
	Doctor's office	Office Inc		
	Artwork	Art store		
	Other			
	Satellite office equipment			
	Computers/monitors (3)	Dell	3,000	
	Printers (3)	Dell	750	
	Routers/communication	Cisco	1,000	
	Phone system	Comdial		3,000
	Phones (7)	Comdial		1,500
	Ultrasound system	GE		
	Subtotal		4,750	4,500
	Sales tax		285	270
	Grand Total		5,035	4,770

Depreciation	Total	Monthly
Pre-2014 additions	$65,000	$5,417
2014 additions	25,000	4,167
Total	$90,000	$9,583

2014 Cost Furniture	Leasehold	Med. Equip	Software	Total	Purchase Date	Comments
	$50,079					
$4,000				4,000	Jul-14	
3,000				3,000	Jul-14	
2,500				2,500	Jul-14	
2,500				2,500	Jul-14	
1,000				1,000	Jul-14	
3,600				3,600	Jul-14	
2,000				2,000	Jul-14	
5,000				5,000	Jul-14	
4,000				4,000	Jul-14	
5,000				5,000	Jul-14	
					Jul-14	
			1,000	4,000	Jul-14	
				750	Jul-14	
				1,000	Jul-14	
				3,000	Jul-14	
				1,500	Jul-14	
		75,000		75,000	Jul-14	
32,600	50,079	75,000	1,000	167,929		
1,956	4,500	60	7,071			
34,556	50,079	79,500	1,060	$175,000		

might purchase an automatic external defibrillator (AED), hoping that using it is not necessary, but making certain it is available if a patient experiences cardiac arrest.

A practice may acquire other assets because they offer a positive economic return to the practice. Use of discounted cash flow techniques helps determine whether a potential investment has an acceptable return on investment (ROI).

The cost of capital equipment or a building is depreciated, or spread over its useful life, according to rules promulgated by GAAP or the Internal Revenue Code. The related depreciation expense will be reflected in the practice's expense budget.

The sample capital budget for Deep South Obstetrics and Gynecology, P.C., is shown in Exhibit 5.2.

Expense Budget (May Incorporate Separate Staff Budget)

The expense budget establishes the anticipated expenses for the practice. It addresses each expense category in the practice, including:

- Support staff salaries and fringe benefits;
- Depreciation and amortization;
- Supplies;
- Occupancy expenses, and;
- Purchased services.

Because much of the expense data depends on production, this budget may only be prepared after completing the related revenue or statistics budget. In preparing the expense budget, the manager needs to consider cost behavior in relationship to volume. Variable costs, such as medical supplies, fluctuate directly with volume. Fixed costs, such as rent, remain the same over a relevant range of activity. (However, be aware that some lease agreements may have growth built in that can change this monthly expense.)

Staff Budget

Some practices prepare a separate staff budget because of the magnitude of medical practice staff salaries in relationship to total overhead. Exhibit 5.3 gives an example of a staff budget. Note that this budget includes projected salary and benefits increases, as well as the addition of staff members when a new physician joins the practice in August.

Exhibit 5.4 shows the expense budget for the hypothetical practice, Deep South Obstetrics and Gynecology, P.C. In anticipation of the new physician's arrival at the practice, this cash basis expense budget includes increased expenditures for medical supplies during July.

Provider Compensation Budget

The provider compensation budget forecasts the amount of profits available to pay or the contractual amounts due to providers. For physician-owned practices, the amount by which practice revenue exceeds the related expenses generally limits the total amount of compensation and other distributions to the physician-owners. The method of distribution varies according to the type of entity and the practice's physician compensation formula. For other types of compensation models, such as RVU or capitation, volume and payer mix will impact the provider compensation budget.

Medical groups that are part of larger integrated delivery systems or are owned by a parent corporation may receive subsidies that can be used to offset operating costs or pay physicians. Accordingly, these organizations need to include both the amount of physician compensation and the amount of operating subsidy in their budgets.

Exhibit 5.5 shows the provider compensation budget for Deep South Obstetrics and Gynecology, P.C. Note that this budget incorporates anticipated bonuses as well as the addition of a physician in August.

Exhibit 5.3
Staff Budget

DEEP SOUTH OBSTETRICS AND GYNECOLOGY, P.C.
Staff Budget — 2014

Pay periods per month					2	2	3
Department/Position	FTE 1-Jan	1-Aug	Name	Hourly Rate	Jan	Feb	Mar
General administrative							
Administrator	1.00	1.00		$43.25	6,920	6,920	10,380
Administrator bonus							
Secretary	1.00	1.00		$12.02	1,923	1,923	2,885
Total general administrative	2.00	2.00			8,843	8,843	13,265
Patient accounting							
Patient accounting manager	1.00	1.00		$19.23	3,077	3,077	4,615
Patient accounting staff	1.00	1.00		$15.00	2,400	2,400	3,600
Patient accounting staff	1.00	1.00		$15.29	2,446	2,446	3,670
Patient accounting staff	1.00	1.00		$15.40	2,464	2,464	3,696
Patient accounting staff	1.00	1.00		$15.85	2,536	2,536	3,804
Total patient accounting	5.00	5.00			12,923	12,923	19,385
Front desk							
Medical receptionists super	1.00	1.00		$16.35	2,616	2,616	3,924
Medical receptionists	1.00	1.00		$12.40	1,984	1,984	2,976
Medical receptionists	1.00	1.00		$12.75	2,040	2,040	3,060
Medical receptionists	1.00	1.00		$13.00	2,080	2,080	3,120
Medical receptionists	1.00	1.00		$12.75	2,040	2,040	3,060
Medical receptionists	1.00	1.00		$13.50	2,160	2,160	3,240
Medical receptionists	1.00	1.00		$13.48	2,157	2,157	3,235
Medical receptionists		1.00		$13.25			
Total front desk	7.00	8.00			15,077	15,077	22,615
Transcription							
Transcriptionists	1.00	1.00		$13.46	2,154	2,154	3,230
Transcriptionists	1.00	1.00		$13.46	2,154	2,154	3,230
Total transcription	2.00	2.00			4,307	4,307	6,461
Medical records							
Medical records supervisor	1.00	1.00		$14.75	2,360	2,360	3,540
Medical records clerk	1.00	1.00		$11.00	1,760	1,760	2,640
Medical records clerk	1.00	1.00		$10.31	1,650	1,650	2,474
Medical records clerk		1.00		$10.50			
Total medical records	3.00	4.00			5,770	5,770	8,654

2	2	2	2	2	3	2	2	2	
Apr	May	Jun	Jul	Aug	Sep	Oct	Nov	Dec	Total
6,920	6,920	6,920	7,197	7,197	10,795	7,197	7,197	7,197	91,759
								10,000	10,000
1,923	1,923	1,923	2,000	2,000	3,000	2,000	2,000	2,000	25,502
8,843	8,843	8,843	9,197	9,197	13,795	9,197	9,197	19,197	127,261
3,077	3,077	3,077	3,200	3,200	4,800	3,200	3,200	3,200	40,798
2,400	2,400	2,400	2,496	2,496	3,744	2,496	2,496	2,496	31,824
2,446	2,446	2,446	2,544	2,544	3,816	2,544	2,544	2,544	32,439
2,464	2,464	2,464	2,563	2,563	3,844	2,563	2,563	2,563	32,673
2,536	2,536	2,536	2,637	2,637	3,956	2,637	2,637	2,637	33,627
12,923	12,923	12,923	13,440	13,440	20,160	13,440	13,440	13,440	171,362
2,616	2,616	2,616	2,721	2,721	4,081	2,721	2,721	2,721	34,688
1,984	1,984	1,984	2,063	2,063	3,095	2,063	2,063	2,063	26,308
2,040	2,040	2,040	2,122	2,122	3,182	2,122	2,122	2,122	27,050
2,080	2,080	2,080	2,163	2,163	3,245	2,163	2,163	2,163	27,581
2,040	2,040	2,040	2,122	2,122	3,182	2,122	2,122	2,122	27,050
2,160	2,160	2,160	2,246	2,246	3,370	2,246	2,246	2,246	28,642
2,157	2,157	2,157	2,243	2,243	3,365	2,243	2,243	2,243	28,599
				2,205	3,307	2,205	2,205	2,205	12,126
15,077	15,077	15,077	15,680	17,885	26,827	17,885	17,885	17,885	212,045
2,154	2,154	2,154	2,240	2,240	3,360	2,240	2,240	2,240	28,557
2,154	2,154	2,154	2,240	2,240	3,360	2,240	2,240	2,240	28,557
4,307	4,307	4,307	4,479	4,479	6,719	4,479	4,479	4,479	57,113
2,360	2,360	2,360	2,454	2,454	3,682	2,454	2,454	2,454	31,294
1,760	1,760	1,760	1,830	1,830	2,746	1,830	1,830	1,830	23,338
1,650	1,650	1,650	1,716	1,716	2,573	1,716	1,716	1,716	21,874
				1,747	2,621	1,747	1,747	1,747	9,610
5,770	5,770	5,770	6,000	7,748	11,621	7,748	7,748	7,748	86,114

Exhibit 5.3
Staff Budget *(continued)*

Pay periods per month					2	2	3
Department/Position	FTE 1-Jan	1-Aug	Name	Hourly Rate	Jan	Feb	Mar
Nursing							
Registered nurse	1.00	1.00		$23.00	3,680	3,680	5,520
Registered nurse	1.00	1.00		$23.76	3,802	3,802	5,702
Registered nurse	1.00	1.00		$22.50	3,600	3,600	5,400
Registered nurse	1.00	1.00		$23.05	3,688	3,688	5,532
Registered nurse		1.00		$23.00			
Licensed practical nurse	1.00	1.00		$16.39	2,622	2,622	3,934
Licensed practical nurse	1.00	1.00		$16.30	2,608	2,608	3,912
Medical assistant	1.00	1.00		$13.00	2,080	2,080	3,120
Medical assistant	1.00	1.00		$12.18	1,949	1,949	2,923
Medical assistant	1.00	1.00		$12.75	2,040	2,040	3,060
Medical assistant	1.00	1.00		$13.50	2,160	2,160	3,240
Medical assistant	1.00	1.00		$13.20	2,112	2,112	3,168
Medical assistant	1.00	1.00		$13.25	2,120	2,120	3,180
Medical assistant		1.00		$13.25			
Total nursing	12.00	14.00			32,461	32,461	48,691
Lab							
Lab tech	1.00	1.00		$12.50	2,000	2,000	3,000
Lab tech part time	0.50	0.50		$12.50	1,000	1,000	1,500
Total lab	1.50	1.50			3,000	3,000	4,500
Ultrasound							
Ultrasound tech supervisor	1.00	1.00		$28.00	4,480	4,480	6,720
Ultrasound tech	1.00	1.00		$22.44	3,590	3,590	5,386
Ultrasound tech	1.00	1.00		$22.00	3,520	3,520	5,280
Ultrasound tech part time	0.50	0.50		$23.40	1,872	1,872	2,808
	3.50	3.50			13,462	13,462	20,194
	36.00	40.00			95,843	95,843	143,765
Payroll Taxes					7,667	7,667	11,501
Employee Benefits							
2013 Monthly benefits costs				16,250	16,250	16,250	16,250
2014 Budgeted increase				7%	1,138	1,138	1,138
2014 Budgeted benefits costs					17,388	17,388	17,388

Budgeted increase eff. July 1   0.04
Add new doctor 7/15/14.
Add satellite office 8/1/14 with 1.00 FTE receptionist, medical records clerk, registered nurse, and medical assistant.

	2	2	2	2	2	3	2	2	2	
	Apr	May	Jun	Jul	Aug	Sep	Oct	Nov	Dec	Total
	3,680	3,680	3,680	3,827	3,827	5,741	3,827	3,827	3,827	48,797
	3,802	3,802	3,802	3,954	3,954	5,930	3,954	3,954	3,954	50,409
	3,600	3,600	3,600	3,744	3,744	5,616	3,744	3,744	3,744	47,736
	3,688	3,688	3,688	3,836	3,836	5,753	3,836	3,836	3,836	48,903
					3,827	5,741	3,827	3,827	3,827	21,050
	2,622	2,622	2,622	2,727	2,727	4,091	2,727	2,727	2,727	34,773
	2,608	2,608	2,608	2,712	2,712	4,068	2,712	2,712	2,712	34,582
	2,080	2,080	2,080	2,163	2,163	3,245	2,163	2,163	2,163	27,581
	1,949	1,949	1,949	2,027	2,027	3,040	2,027	2,027	2,027	25,841
	2,040	2,040	2,040	2,122	2,122	3,182	2,122	2,122	2,122	27,050
	2,160	2,160	2,160	2,246	2,246	3,370	2,246	2,246	2,246	28,642
	2,112	2,112	2,112	2,196	2,196	3,295	2,196	2,196	2,196	28,005
	2,120	2,120	2,120	2,205	2,205	3,307	2,205	2,205	2,205	28,111
					2,205	3,307	2,205	2,205	2,205	12,126
	32,461	32,461	32,461	33,759	39,791	59,687	39,791	39,791	39,791	463,606
	2,000	2,000	2,000	2,080	2,080	3,120	2,080	2,080	2,080	26,520
	1,000	1,000	1,000	2,080	2,080	3,120	2,080	2,080	2,080	20,020
	3,000	3,000	3,000	4,160	4,160	6,240	4,160	4,160	4,160	46,540
	4,480	4,480	4,480	4,659	4,659	6,989	4,659	4,659	4,659	59,405
	3,590	3,590	3,590	3,734	3,734	5,601	3,734	3,734	3,734	47,609
	3,520	3,520	3,520	3,661	3,661	5,491	3,661	3,661	3,661	46,675
	1,872	1,872	1,872	3,894	3,894	5,841	3,894	3,894	3,894	37,477
	13,462	13,462	13,462	15,948	15,948	23,922	15,948	15,948	15,948	191,166
	95,843	95,843	95,843	102,664	112,648	168,972	112,648	112,648	122,648	1,355,208
	7,667	7,667	7,667	8,213	9,012	13,518	9,012	9,012	9,812	108,417
	16,250	16,250	16,250	18,055	18,055	18,055	18,055	18,055	18,055	205,830
	1,138	1,138	1,138	1,264	1,264	1,264	1,264	1,264	1,264	14,408
	17,388	17,388	17,388	19,319	19,319	19,319	19,319	19,319	19,319	220,238

Exhibit 5.4
Expense Budget

DEEP SOUTH OBSTETRICS AND GYNECOLOGY, P.C.

Expense Budget — 2014

	Jan	Feb	Mar	Apr	May	Jun
Services and General Expenses						
Malpractice insurance	$80,000			$80,000		
Medical and surgical supplies	15,000	15,000	15,000	15,000	15,000	15,000
Depreciation	5,417	5,417	5,417	5,417	5,417	5,417
Amortization	417	417	417	417	417	417
Rent	27,500	27,500	27,500	27,500	27,500	27,500
Information technology	7,500	7,500	7,500	7,500	7,500	7,500
Other general and administrative exp.	13,500	13,500	13,500	13,500	13,500	13,500
Total services and general expenses	$149,334	$69,334	$69,334	$149,334	$69,334	$69,334

Master Budget

The master budget brings together the practice's various budgets in either formal or informal financial statement formats. The master budget in Exhibit 5.6 gives the income statement amounts from the various budgets by month. The master budget in Exhibit 5.7 shows the annual budget amounts compared to the prior year actual, computes the variance, indicates the source budget, and provides an explanation of significant changes.

Cash Budget

The cash budget is the cornerstone for short-term cash management in a practice. It provides management with a forecast of the organization's short-term availability of cash, its need for supplemental cash in the form of a loan or line of credit to meet predicted expenses, and any periods with excess cash available for short-term investments.

Jul	Aug	Sep	Oct	Nov	Dec	Total	Comments
$100,000			$100,000			$360,000	Quarterly quote
20,000	16,000	17,000	17,000	17,000	17,000	194,000	
9,583	9,583	9,583	9,583	9,583	9,583	90,000	
459	459	459	459	459	459	5,256	
31,700	31,700	31,700	31,700	31,700	31,700	355,200	
8,500	8,500	8,500	8,500	8,500	8,500	96,000	
13,500	13,500	13,500	13,500	13,500	13,500	162,000	
$183,742	$79,742	$80,742	$180,742	$80,742	$80,742	$1,262,456	

Exhibit 5.8 shows the monthly cash budget for the hypothetical practice, Deep South Obstetrics and Gynecology, P.C. Because this practice is a cash basis practice, its cash budget requires only a few adjustments to translate net income per the operating budget to projected cash flow. Accrual basis practices usually have more differences between operating net income and cash flow. An alternate approach is the direct method, which itemizes cash receipts and disbursements rather than reconciling them to net income.

Departmental Budget

Larger practices or those with multiple locations, service lines, and/ or specialties often prepare separate budgets for each department. These departmental budgets are then combined to form the organization's master budget.

Exhibit 5.5
Provider Compensation Budget

DEEP SOUTH OBSTETRICS AND GYNECOLOGY, P.C.
Provider Compensation Budget – 2014

Physician/Extender	Jan	Feb	Mar	Apr	May	Jun
Base Salary						
Smith	15,000	15,000	15,000	15,000	15,000	15,000
Jones	15,000	15,000	15,000	15,000	15,000	15,000
Harris	16,667	16,667	16,667	16,667	16,667	16,667
Thruman	16,667	16,667	16,667	16,667	16,667	16,667
Dunn	16,667	16,667	16,667	16,667	16,667	16,667
Thompson	16,667	16,667	16,667	16,667	16,667	16,667
Cohen	16,667	16,667	16,667	16,667	16,667	16,667
New doctor						
Total physicians	113,335	113,335	113,335	113,335	113,335	113,335
Bonuses						200,000
Grand total physicians	113,335	113,335	113,335	113,335	113,335	313,335
Physician payroll tax %	7.6%	7.6%	7.6%	7.6%	6.0%	1.4%
Physician payroll tax $	8,613	8,613	8,613	8,613	6,800	4,387
Physician benefits	34,000	34,000	34,000	34,000	34,000	34,000
Physician extenders						
Base Salary						
Bence	4,792	4,792	4,792	4,792	4,792	4,792
Davis	4,792	4,792	4,792	4,792	4,792	4,792
Starr	5,000	5,000	5,000	5,000	5,000	5,000
Total	14,584	14,584	14,584	14,584	14,584	14,584
Bonuses						10,000
Grand Total Extenders	14,584	14,584	14,584	14,584	14,584	24,584
Extenders payroll tax %	8.0%	8.0%	8.0%	8.0%	8.0%	8.0%
Extenders payroll tax $	1,167	1,167	1,167	1,167	1,167	1,967
Extenders benefits	3,000	3,000	3,000	3,000	3,000	3,000

Jul	Aug	Sep	Oct	Nov	Dec	Total
15,000	15,000	15,000	15,000	15,000	15,000	180,000
15,000	15,000	15,000	15,000	15,000	15,000	180,000
16,667	16,667	16,667	16,667	16,667	16,667	200,004
16,667	16,667	16,667	16,667	16,667	16,667	200,004
16,667	16,667	16,667	16,667	16,667	16,667	200,004
16,667	16,667	16,667	16,667	16,667	16,667	200,004
16,667	16,667	16,667	16,667	16,667	16,667	200,004
12,500	12,500	12,500	12,500	12,500	12,500	75,000
125,835	125,835	125,835	125,835	125,835	125,835	1,435,020
					200,000	400,000
125,835	125,835	125,835	125,835	125,835	325,835	1,835,020
2.0%	2.0%	2.0%	2.0%	2.0%	2.0%	
2,517	2,517	2,517	2,517	2,517	6,517	64,741
37,000	37,000	37,000	37,000	37,000	37,000	426,000
4,792	4,792	4,792	4,792	4,792	4,792	57,504
4,792	4,792	4,792	4,792	4,792	4,792	57,504
5,000	5,000	5,000	5,000	5,000	5,000	60,000
14,584	14,584	14,584	14,584	14,584	14,584	175,008
					15,000	25,000
14,584	14,584	14,584	14,584	14,584	29,584	200,008
8.0%	8.0%	8.0%	8.0%	8.0%	8.0%	
1,167	1,167	1,167	1,167	1,167	2,367	16,001
3,000	3,000	3,000	3,000	3,000	3,000	36,000

Exhibit 5.6
Master Budget by Month

DEEP SOUTH OBSTETRICS AND GYNECOLOGY, P.C.
Master Budget by Month – 2014

	Jan	Feb	Mar	Apr	May
Charges	844,600	705,550	880,650	849,750	870,350
Revenues:					
Net fee-for-service revenue	409,981	417,285	417,785	402,512	456,576
Capitation revenue					
Other	23,750	21,750	24,750	22,750	24,750
Net revenue	433,731	439,035	442,535	425,262	481,326
Operating Expenses					
Salaries and benefits					
Staff salaries	95,843	95,843	143,765	95,843	95,843
Payroll taxes	7,667	7,667	11,501	7,667	7,667
Employee benefits	17,388	17,388	17,388	17,388	17,388
Total salaries and benefits	120,898	120,898	172,653	120,898	120,898
Services and General Expenses					
Malpractice insurance	80,000	–	–	80,000	–
Medical and surgical supplies	15,000	15,000	15,000	15,000	15,000
Depreciation	5,417	5,417	5,417	5,417	5,417
Amortization	417	417	417	417	417
Rent	27,500	27,500	27,500	27,500	27,500
Information technology	7,500	7,500	7,500	7,500	7,500
Other general and administrative exp.	13,500	13,500	13,500	13,500	13,500
Total services and general expenses	149,334	69,334	69,334	149,334	69,334
Provider-related expenses					
Physician salaries	113,335	113,335	113,335	113,335	113,335
Physician payroll taxes	8,613	8,613	8,613	8,613	6,800
Physician benefits	34,000	34,000	34,000	34,000	34,000
Total physician costs	155,948	155,948	155,948	155,948	154,135
Nurse practitioner salaries	14,584	14,584	14,584	14,584	14,584
Nurse practitioner payroll taxes	1,167	1,167	1,167	1,167	1,167
Nurse practitioner benefits	3,000	3,000	3,000	3,000	3,000
Total nurse practitioner costs	18,751	18,751	18,751	18,751	18,751
Total provider costs	174,699	174,699	174,699	174,699	172,886
Total Operating Expenses	444,931	364,931	416,687	444,931	363,118
Income from Operations	(11,200)	74,103	25,848	(19,670)	118,208
Nonmedical costs					
Interest and taxes	750	750	750	750	750
Income (Loss)	(11,950)	73,353	25,098	(20,420)	117,458

Jun	Jul	Aug	Sep	Oct	Nov	Dec	Total
829,150	777,650	828,400	874,300	945,800	894,000	863,400	10,163,600
449,818	449,278	425,760	417,512	443,260	472,056	486,934	5,248,756
23,750	22,750	22,750	24,750	24,750	23,750	21,750	282,000
473,568	472,028	448,510	442,262	468,010	495,806	508,684	5,530,756
95,843	102,664	112,648	168,972	112,648	112,648	122,648	1,355,208
7,667	8,213	9,012	13,518	9,012	9,012	9,812	108,417
17,388	19,319	19,319	19,319	19,319	19,319	19,319	220,238
120,898	130,196	140,978	201,808	140,978	140,978	151,778	1,683,862
–	100,000	–	–	100,000	–	–	360,000
15,000	20,000	16,000	17,000	17,000	17,000	17,000	194,000
5,417	9,583	9,583	9,583	9,583	9,583	9,583	90,000
417	459	459	459	459	459	459	5,256
27,500	31,700	31,700	31,700	31,700	31,700	31,700	355,200
7,500	8,500	8,500	8,500	8,500	8,500	8,500	96,000
13,500	13,500	13,500	13,500	13,500	13,500	13,500	162,000
69,334	183,742	79,742	80,742	180,742	80,742	80,742	1,262,456
313,335	125,835	125,835	125,835	125,835	125,835	325,835	1,835,020
4,387	2,517	2,517	2,517	2,517	2,517	6,517	64,741
34,000	37,000	37,000	37,000	37,000	37,000	37,000	426,000
351,722	165,352	165,352	165,352	165,352	165,352	369,352	2,325,761
24,584	14,584	14,584	14,584	14,584	14,584	29,584	200,008
1,967	1,167	1,167	1,167	1,167	1,167	2,367	16,001
3,000	3,000	3,000	3,000	3,000	3,000	3,000	36,000
29,551	18,751	18,751	18,751	18,751	18,751	34,951	252,009
381,272	184,102	184,102	184,102	184,102	184,102	404,302	2,577,769
571,505	498,040	404,823	466,653	505,823	405,823	636,823	5,524,088
(97,936)	(26,013)	43,687	(24,391)	(37,813)	89,983	(128,139)	6,668
750	750	750	750	750	750	750	9,000
(98,686)	(26,763)	42,937	(25,141)	(38,563)	89,233	(128,889)	(2,332)

Exhibit 5.7
Master Budget by Year

DEEP SOUTH OBSTETRICS AND GYNECOLOGY, P.C.
Master Budget – 2014

	Source	Actual 2013
Charges	Revenue Budget	$9,620,000
Revenues:		
Net fee-for-service revenue	Revenue Budget	$4,980,000
Capitation revenue	Revenue Budget	
Other	Revenue Budget	270,000
Net revenue		5,250,000
Operating Expenses		
Salaries and benefits		
Staff salaries	Staff Budget	1,246,000
Payroll taxes	Staff Budget	100,000
Employee benefits	Staff Budget	195,000
Total salaries and benefits		1,541,000
Services and General Expenses		
Malpractice insurance	Expense Budget	310,000
Medical and surgical supplies	Expense Budget	173,000
Depreciation	Expense Budget	75,000
Amortization	Expense Budget	5,000
Rent	Expense Budget	330,000
Information technology	Expense Budget	90,000
Other general and administrative exp.	Expense Budget	157,000
Total services and general expenses		1,140,000
Provider-related expenses		
Physician salaries	Provider Comp. Budget	1,865,000
Physician payroll taxes	Provider Comp. Budget	60,000
Physician benefits	Provider Comp. Budget	390,000
Total physician costs	Provider Comp. Budget	2,315,000
Nurse practitioner salaries	Provider Comp. Budget	196,000
Nurse practitioner payroll taxes	Provider Comp. Budget	15,600
Nurse practitioner benefits	Provider Comp. Budget	33,400
Total nurse practitioner costs	Provider Comp. Budget	245,000
Total provider costs	Provider Comp. Budget	2,560,000
Total Operating Expenses		5,241,000
Income from Operations		9,000
Nonmedical costs		
Interest and taxes		(10,000)
Income (Loss)		($1,000)

Budget 2014	Variance $	%	
$10,163,600	$543,600	5.7%	Growth and new doctor 7/14
5,248,756	268,756	5.4%	Growth and new doctor 7/14
282,000	12,000	4.4%	Growth of contract ultrasounds
5,530,756	280,756	5.3%	
1,355,208	109,208	8.8%	New staff for new office 8/14
108,417	8,417	8.4%	New staff for new office 8/15
220,238	25,238	12.9%	New staff and higher health costs
1,683,862	142,862	9.3%	
360,000	50,000	16.1%	Malpractice increases per quote and new doctor
194,000	21,000	12.1%	New office and more contract ultrasounds
90,000	15,000	20.0%	New office
5,256	256	5.1%	
355,200	25,200	7.6%	New office
96,000	6,000	6.7%	New office
162,000	5,000	3.2%	
1,262,456	122,456	10.7%	
1,835,020	(29,980)	−1.6%	Lower bonuses lower to fund new doctor start-up
64,741	4,741	7.9%	New doctor
426,000	36,000	9.2%	New doctor and health increases
2,325,761	10,761	0.5%	
200,008	4,008	2.0%	Annual increases
16,001	401	2.6%	Annual increases
36,000	2,600	7.8%	Health increases
252,009	7,009	2.9%	
2,577,769	17,769	0.7%	
5,524,088	283,088	5.4%	
6,668	(2,332)	−25.9%	
(9,000)	1,000	−10.0%	
($2,332)	($1,332)	133.2%	

Exhibit 5.8
Cash Budget

DEEP SOUTH OBSTETRICS AND GYNECOLOGY, P.C.
Cash Budget – 2014

	Jan	Feb	Mar	Apr	May
Net Income(loss)	($11,950)	$73,353	$25,098	($20,420)	$117,458
Add back					
Depreciation	5,417	5,417	5,417	5,417	5,417
Amortization	417	417	417	417	417
Retirement accrual	25,000	25,000	25,000	25,000	25,000
Long-term debt proceeds					
Total Adds	30,834	30,834	30,834	30,834	30,834
Subtract					
Principal payments	(2,000)	(1,950)	(1,900)	(1,850)	(1,800)
Retirement contribution			(300,000)		
Equipment purchases					
Total Subtracts	(2,000)	(1,950)	(301,900)	(1,850)	(1,800)
Cash flow for month	16,884	102,237	(245,968)	8,564	146,492
Cash, beginning of month	110,000	126,884	229,121	(16,847)	(8,282)
Cash, end of month	$126,884	$229,121	($16,847)	($8,282)	$138,210

Budget Methodologies

There is no one best way to prepare a budget, but there are many useful templates you can use depending on what purpose the budget needs to serve.

Fixed vs. Flexible

A fixed budget computes one best estimate for revenues and related expenses. Budget variances are based on differences between actual performance and the estimated set of numbers.

A flexible budget assumes that actual results may vary and provides a mechanism for computing budget variances at different volume levels,

Jun	Jul	Aug	Sep	Oct	Nov	Dec	Total
($98,686)	($26,763)	$42,937	($25,141)	($38,563)	$89,233	($128,889)	($2,332)
5,417	9,583	9,583	9,583	9,583	9,583	9,583	90,000
417	459	459	459	459	459	459	5,256
25,000	25,000	25,000	25,000	25,000	25,000	25,000	300,000
	140,000						140,000
30,834	175,042	35,042	35,042	35,042	35,042	35,042	535,256
(1,750)	(1,700)	(1,650)	(1,600)	(1,550)	(1,500)	(1,450)	(20,700)
							(300,000)
	(175,000)						(175,000)
(1,750)	(176,700)	(1,650)	(1,600)	(1,550)	(1,500)	(1,450)	(495,700)
(69,602)	(28,421)	76,329	8,301	(5,071)	122,775	(95,297)	37,224
138,210	68,608	40,187	116,516	124,817	119,746	242,521	
$68,608	$40,187	$116,516	$124,817	$119,746	$242,521	$147,224	

based on a careful assessment of fixed, step-fixed, and variable costs. The advantage of a flexible budget is its ability to better assess financial performance at different activity levels. The primary disadvantage is that it is more time consuming.

Traditional vs. Zero Based

The traditional budget process uses prior and current-year activity levels, revenues, and expenses as a basis for determining prospective values for the coming year. Conversely, zero-based budgeting begins each budget without considering past performance. Essentially, the budget starts at zero and all budget assumptions are reassessed.

187

The primary disadvantage of zero-based budgeting is that it is more time consuming than traditional budgeting, With the lack of historic basis you lose the advantage of trending data. The major advantage is that, because the zero-based budget process forces a practice to start over, it provides more insights into practice revenues and expenses. Thus, the practice will be more likely to set up its business in such a manner that by meeting its budget objectives it will also be successful in achieving its strategic or business plan.

Common Budget Pitfalls

Practices sometimes sabotage a budget's potential effectiveness by taking too little time to complete the budgeting process, using numbers that are unreliable, and underestimating or overestimating expenses and targets.

Failure to Allow Enough Time

Practice leaders should begin the budget process early enough to allow enough time to get good numbers. It is also important to develop a comprehensive schedule identifying when all the necessary components are due along with the responsible party. This can involve time to rework the initial numbers if they are inconsistent with each other or with the practice's operational and strategic goals.

Overreliance on Historical Data

Although prior-year amounts and other historical data are often useful in estimating budget amounts, practices need to avoid relying too heavily on retrospective data. Those involved in the budget process need to consider how known and anticipated changes in the practice and the marketplace in general will affect these amounts. For example, changes in fee schedules, payer mix, and the local economy impact net revenues. The addition of a physician or a new location will impact revenues, as well as many costs. The budget should address inflation and significant increases in costs, such as employee health insurance.

Budgetary Slack

Managers sometimes hedge against adversity by submitting easily obtainable budget amounts, especially when personnel evaluations are largely based on adhering to the budget or when across-the-board cost reductions are anticipated.[2] One estimate holds that for traditionally managed organizations, the cost of inefficiency and waste is between 20 percent and 40 percent of the budget.[3]

The danger here is that budgetary slack misleads leaders about the true potential of the practice. To guard against budgetary slack, administrators may benchmark submitted budget amounts against industry data. Zero-based budgeting (discussed earlier in this chapter) may also reduce the potential for budgetary slack.

Finally, budget personnel need to consider whether historical numbers reflect waste and inefficiencies that can be improved in the next budget cycle.

Unattainable Budgets

While slack budgets rarely challenge managers, overly ambitious or even unobtainable budgets fail to motivate and ultimately lead to further disengagement. Because they offer little opportunity to avoid failure, unattainable budgets are more likely to increase anxiety than stimulate motivation or creative thinking. If using unrealistic projections, practice personnel will not take the budget process seriously, and the organization will not reap many of the potential benefits from the process.

Best Bet: The Challenging but Attainable Budget

Research indicates that budgets which are challenging but attainable improve performance. Jack Welch, the legendary former chief executive officer of General Electric, agrees: He claims that challenging budgets energize and motivate managers, unleashing creative, out-of-the-box thinking.[4]

Depreciation

Practices often acquire long-term assets in the course of their business operations. Although these assets have expected useful lives of greater than one year, most of these assets (other than land) will not last forever.

The practice needs a mechanism for spreading the cost of these assets over their expected useful lives; this mechanism is *depreciation*. During each year of the asset's estimated life, the practice recognizes a portion of the asset's cost as an expense and reduces the net value of the asset on the balance sheet accordingly.

Although various methods for computing depreciation exist, the method a practice uses depends largely on its method of accounting and applicable tax rules at the time.

Straight-Line Depreciation

Straight-line depreciation spreads an asset's cost evenly over its expected useful life. If related revenue flows are somewhat constant during this period, this method is appropriate.

Accelerated Depreciation Methods

Accelerated depreciation methods expend larger amounts of the asset cost in the early years of the asset's life and correspondingly lower amounts in later years. The *double-declining balance method* recognizes depreciation at twice the straight-line rate based on the asset's *book value* (cost less accumulated depreciation). The *150 percent declining balance method* recognizes depreciation at one and one-half times the straight-line rate based on the asset's book value. The *sum-of-the-year's digits method* computes a decreasing amount of depreciation each year using the fractions obtained by the sum of the digits in the number of years of an asset's life. For example, the depreciation of an asset with an estimated useful life of five years is: 5/ (5 + 4 + 3 + 2 + 1) or 5/15 the first year, 4/15 the second year, and so on.

An accelerated depreciation method makes economic sense when the bulk of an asset's production comes in the early years of its life, thus better matching expenses with the related revenue.

Units-of-Production Depreciation

The *units-of-production* method of depreciation expenses the production for the year as a percentage of the total expected production during the asset's life. This depreciation method was developed to ensure matching an asset's expense with the revenue generated. It is appropriate when the practice expects an asset's production to vary during its useful life.

Tax Depreciation

Income tax rules generally allow the use of accelerated depreciation methods for tangible personal property, such as medical and office equipment. Allowable methods under the General Depreciation System version of the Modified Accelerated Cost Recovery System allow for a 200 percent or 150 percent declining balance method that switches to straight-line depreciation when this amount provides a greater or equal deduction.[5] In recent years, tax laws have allowed qualifying taxpayers to expense the cost of qualifying asset additions up to a certain dollar amount in the year of acquisition. This is referred to as a *Section 179 deduction*. Recent laws have also provided for bonus depreciation on certain assets. Many practices have taken advantage of these accelerated methods to save income taxes.

In addition to specifying certain depreciation methods, the tax laws contain guidance as to the useful lives for various types of assets. This information is available in *Publication 946: How to Depreciate Property* from the Internal Revenue Service.[6]

Book vs. Tax Depreciation

Although tax rules generally permit all qualifying taxpayers to take accelerated depreciation on applicable assets, GAAP requires that depreciation be economically reasonable; consequently, many accrual basis practices use a less aggressive depreciation method for book purposes. Differing book and tax depreciation methods contribute to the potential for deferred income taxes on accrual basis balance sheets.

Because cash method practices often use the same depreciation method for book purposes that they use for income tax purposes, the depreciation expense and resulting net income amounts reported on the practice's financial statements may fluctuate significantly. Although accelerated methods may not represent economic reality, they are allowable for tax purposes and usually reduce a practice's income tax liability. Consequently, practices generally use them for tax purposes.

Financial Accounting vs. Management Accounting

Although financial accounting deals with external reporting to parties such as creditors, management accounting focuses on providing information to management for internal decision-making.

Financial accounting must comply with specific external guidelines, such as GAAP or OCBOA. This ensures that the practice's financial statements are comparable with financial statements produced by other entities, so that an external party who is knowledgeable in financial reporting will understand the financial statements. The entries in a practice's general ledger generally conform to the basis of accounting that the practice uses for financial reporting purposes.

Unlike financial accounting, management accounting does not have a strict set of guidelines. Although accounting textbooks suggest approaches for providing this information, these approaches are not requirements. An organization has the flexibility to provide its management accounting information in the manner that best facilitates its internal decision making.

Cost Accounting

Cost accounting "measures and reports financial and nonfinancial information relating to the cost of acquiring or utilizing resources in an organization."[7] It supplies information for both financial accounting and management accounting.[8] Although administrators sometimes use the term *cost accounting* to refer to cost allocation, the field of cost accounting is much more comprehensive. Cost accounting textbooks usually include numerous other topics, such as budgets and projections, inventory management, computing return on investment, and short-term decision making.

Short-Term Decision Making

The cost accounting model for short-term decision making is cost volume-profit analysis, which includes break-even analysis. To understand this model, one must first understand cost behavior, including the difference between fixed and variable costs and how changes in volume affect these costs. By analyzing how changes in fixed costs, variable cost per unit, price per unit, and volume affect profit, cost-volume-profit analysis seeks to answer the question, "What if?" The components of cost-volume-profit analysis can form an algebraic equation that determines a practice's break-even point.

Cost Behavior: Fixed vs. Variable Costs

Fixed costs remain the same in total during a period, despite a large range of potential activity (referred to as the *relevant range*). For example, a practice's rent expense generally remains the same whether the physicians see no patients or have a packed schedule.

Exhibit 5.9 The Cost-Volume-Profit Analysis Variables	
Variable	**Example of Changes**
Selling price	Change in payer fee schedule Improved collection of copayments
Volume	Increase in number of patients Increase in number of procedures per patient
Variable cost per unit	Decrease in cost of medical supplies (i.e., from getting competitive bids) Increase in cost of linen service
Fixed cost	Increase in rent Decrease in malpractice insurance (i.e., from finding a new carrier)

Exhibit 5.10

The Cost-Volume-Profit Formula

Financial accounting model	Revenues – Expenses = Profit
Basic cost-volume-profit model	Revenues – Fixed Costs – Variable Costs = Profit
Cost-volume-profit formula	(Volume × Sales Price per Unit) – Fixed Costs – (Volume × Variable Costs per Unit) = Profit

Exhibit 5.11

Contribution Margin

Contribution Margin	Formula
Contribution margin per unit	Selling Price per Unit – Variable Cost per Unit
Contribution percentage	(Selling Price per Unit – Variable Cost per Unit)/ Selling Price per Unit
Total contribution margin	Total Selling Price – Total Variable Costs

Exhibit 5.12

Break-Even Analysis Formula

Break-Even Point	Formula
In units	BEPQ = FC/CMU
In net revenues	BEPR = FC/CM%

Definitions:

BEPQ = break-even point in quantity
BEPR = break-even point in net revenues
FC = total fixed costs
CMU = contribution margin per unit
CM% = contribution margin percentage

Other examples of fixed costs include malpractice insurance and certain staff costs, such as the administrator's base salary.

Variable costs vary directly with the practice's volume. For example, a practice's medical supplies expense generally increases in proportion to its volume. Suppose a practice's medical supplies cost runs $1 per office visit. If the practice sees no patients, it incurs no medical supplies expense. If it sees 1,000 patients, it incurs $1,000 medical supplies expense; if it sees 10,000 patients, it incurs $10,000 medical supplies expense, and so on.

A hybrid type of cost is the *step-fixed cost*. These costs remain the same over various ranges of activity, but increase by discrete amounts, or *steps*, as the level of activity changes from one range to the next. Many staff costs are step-fixed costs.

Cost-Volume-Profit Analysis

Cost-volume-profit analysis studies the effect that changes in volume, selling price per unit, variable cost per unit, and fixed costs have on revenues, costs, and net income from operations. Exhibit 5.9 provides examples of changes in each of these variables. Using these variables, the income statement equation can be restated as a cost-volume-profit formula. See Exhibit 5.10.

Note that the total revenues and the total variable costs both depend on volume, whereas fixed costs remain the same regardless of the volume. This means that for each additional unit of volume, the bottom line will change by the difference between the sales price per unit and the variable cost per unit. This amount is called the contribution margin; it can be expressed as either an amount per unit, a percentage, or in total.

After volume reaches a certain level, the total contribution margin is sufficient to cover the fixed costs (Exhibit 5.11). This level is called the *break-even point*. After reaching the break-even point, each additional unit of volume creates incremental profit equal to the contribution margin per unit.

Exhibit 5.13
Big Valley Radiology Break-Even Analysis Example

Big Valley Radiology has experienced a 1.5 percent Medicare cut. Because its other payers benchmark off Medicare, this cut affects all of its reimbursement. The following table shows the practice's summary financial information before and after the cut.

Description	Before	Change	After
Net Revenue	$5,000,000	($75,000)	$4,925,000
Fixed Overhead	1,570,000		1,570,000
Variable Overhead	280,000		280,000
Total Amount Distributable to Physicians	3,150,000	(75,000)	3,075,000
Profitability per Physician	$450,000	(10,714)	$439,286
Number of Procedures	110,000		110,000
Number of FTE physicians	7		7

Note that this is a change in sales price (reimbursement). Because the practice's volume was unaffected, variable costs remain the same in total. In computing revised break-even analysis, the decrease in sales price (reimbursement) decreased the contribution margin.

Description	Before	Change	After
Contribution Margin	$4,720,000	(75,000)	$4,645,000
Contribution Margin per Unit	$42.91	($0.68)	$42.23
Contribution Margin Percentage	94.40%	($0.08)	94.32%

Conducting break-even analyses helps a practice understand its current financial structure and facilitates short-term decision making. The break-even point can be computed in either units or in net revenues (Exhibit 5.12).

A practice can use break-even analyses to compute the volume or net revenues required to achieve certain levels of profit by increasing fixed costs by the amount of desired profit.

Exhibit 5.13

Big Valley Radiology Break-Even Analysis Example *(continued)*

Computing Break-Even Point in Quantity

The following example uses break-even analysis to compute the number of additional procedures the group must perform to maintain the same profitability per FTE physician it had prior to the increase.

BEPQ = FC/CMU

(Break-Even Point in Quantity = Fixed Costs/Contribution Margin per Unit)

- Fixed Costs = Desired profitability + Fixed Overhead
    $3,150,000 + $1,570,000 = $4,720,000
- CMU = RU – VCU
    Contribution Margin per Unit = Revenue per Unit – Variable Cost per Unit)
    - Revenue per Unit = $4,925,000/110,000 = $44.77
    - Variable Cost per Unit = $280,000/110,000 = $2.54
- CMU = $44.77 – $2.54 = $42.23

BEPQ = $4,720,000 /$42.23 = 111,769

The group must perform 1,769 more procedures to make up for the Medicare cuts.

Computing Break-Even Point in Revenues

The following example uses break-even analysis to compute the additional revenue level the group must achieve to maintain the same profitability per FTE physician it had prior to the Medicare pay cut.

BEPR = FC/CM%

(Break-Even Point in Revenues = Fixed Costs/Contribution Margin %)

- Fixed Costs = Desired Profitability + Fixed Overhead
    $4,720,000 (same as preceding example)
- Contribution Margin % = Contribution Margin per Unit/Revenue per Unit
    $42.23/ $44.77 = 94.32%

BEPR = $4,720,000 / 0.9432 = $5,004,241

The group needs to increase its revenues $79,241 to make up for the 1.5% Medicare (and total reimbursement) cut.

The case study in Exhibit 5.13 illustrates break-even and cost volume-profit analysis for a hypothetical radiology practice, Big Valley Radiology.[9]

Exhibit 5.14 displays break-even analysis for Big Valley Radiology in graph form. The arrow indicates the profit range.

Exhibit 5.14
Break-Even Analysis for Big Valley Radiology

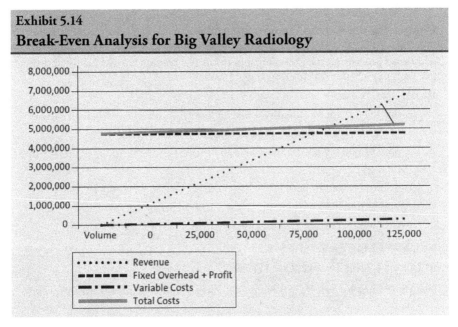

Break-Even Analysis under Capitation

The preceding discussion assumes the practice is compensated based on fee-for-service (FFS) or discounted FFS contracts. When practice revenues are derived from capitation, the amount of revenue is no longer based on volume of services provided. Capitation revenue is computed on the number of members for which the practice is responsible regardless of the services provided to the members. The actual revenue under capitation is the number of members for the month times the "per member per month" rate. Like fixed costs, capitated revenues remain the same regardless of volume. Thus, for capitation, the only variable that changes with volume is variable costs. Hence, the capitation model is profitable until variable costs increase to the point that they exceed net revenues, less fixed costs.

Exhibit 5.15 shows the break-even graph for Big Valley Radiology assuming all revenue is capitated.

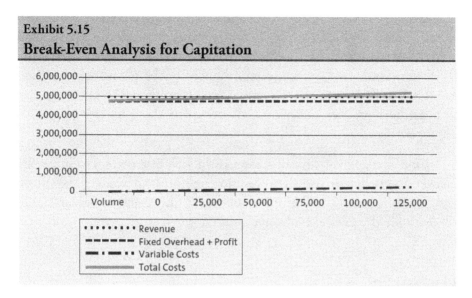

Exhibit 5.15
Break-Even Analysis for Capitation

Legend:
- Revenue
- Fixed Overhead + Profit
- Variable Costs
- Total Costs

Cost Allocation

Sometimes obtaining the information necessary to facilitate economic decision making requires cost allocation. For example, a practice may allocate costs to help determine whether a specific location is profitable, evaluate a proposed contract, or set its fee schedule. Many physician compensation plans require cost allocation.

A popular cost accounting textbook defines *cost allocation* as the "assignment of indirect costs to a particular cost object"[10] and a *cost object* as "anything for which a measurement of costs is desired."[11] Direct costs are those that can be traced to a cost object in a cost effective manner. Conversely, indirect costs cannot be traced to a particular cost object in a cost-effective manner.[12]

For example, in computing the profit or loss for a satellite office, an administrator can easily trace the rent for that office and the salaries of its employees to that particular satellite office. These expenses are considered direct costs. The costs of a central administrative office pertain to multiple locations and cannot be easily traced to a particular clinic; these are indirect costs that must be allocated.

Cost accounting textbooks contain many different cost accounting models, some of which are quite complex. The best model for a particular situation depends on the industry, the attributes of the business and its owners, and the facts and circumstances of the particular situation. Exhibit 5.16 lists some of the methods commonly used to allocate costs in a medical practice and situations in which these models might be appropriate.

One challenge of cost allocation is the lack of a correct or incorrect answer to each scenario. The decision requires an understanding of cost allocation methodology, cost behavior, the specific problem, and the individual practice. It also requires judgment and a commitment to fairness.

Managing Investments

A medical group's governing body and financial manager are faced with many investment decisions, some with long-range implications and others affecting the immediate future. Usually the approach involves measuring the benefits to be achieved from an alternative and comparing those with the costs of pursuing that course of action. A crucial element, then, is to identify, measure, and compare benefits and costs attributable to each kind of decision. Most of these decisions, within an investment context, should be treated as an evaluation process that compares alternative avenues for placing some of a medical group's assets into ventures to achieve some amount of return.

There are two general classifications of these investment alternatives, and each type requires considerably different information for analysis. The first type — *long range* — involves the acquisition or replacement of capacity and requires a long period of time before the benefits are fully realized. These investments normally entail acquiring buildings, equipment, and, to some extent, key people. The second type of investment alternative — *short range* — embodies the use of capacity, usually within a short period of time.

Exhibit 5.16
Cost Allocation Methods in a Medical Practice

Method	Situation in Which This Method Might Be Appropriate
Square footage	Allocating rent and utility costs to departments
Full-time equivalent count	Allocating human resource management department costs
Payroll costs	Allocating workers' compensation insurance costs
Percentage of revenues	Allocating billing costs to divisions or locations
Volume — may be measured by number of procedures, charges, or relative value units	Allocating variable costs such as medical supplies, linens, and scheduling costs
Usage	Allocating information technology department costs based on the number of computers
Stipulated or agreed-on percentage	Based on compromise or agreement among the group, particularly when no one method clearly reflects economic reality — for example, a practice might allocate a specific percentage of fixed expenses to a part-time physician
	For simplification — for example, a practice may assign administrative costs to individual clinics based on a stipulated percentage for interim purposes

Long-Range Investment Decisions

Long-range investments are commitments of funds to acquire an asset that will provide benefits over a long period of time. Such investments for a medical group pertain to acquiring buildings, purchasing equipment, and leasing facilities or equipment. In all these cases, there is an addition to or a replacement of the capacity of the group in the form of long-lived assets to render medical services.

Short-Range Investment Decisions

Short-range decisions differ from long-range decisions in three primary areas. First, as the name implies, short-range decisions relate to short periods of time. Although the time value of money is important for long-range decisions, it is not critical in short-range decisions and is generally not considered in the analysis.

The *time value of money* means that a unit of money — the dollar — is worth more today by having it in hand than it is worth at some point in the future because of the need to consider the interest factor or a return for the use of money. This is true because short-term decisions usually involve a limited investment in and a quick recovery of cash. Second, short-range decisions usually involve repetitive activities, while long-range choices may not. Because the immediate future will likely be similar to the recent past, accounting measurements of revenue and costs are relevant for short-term analysis. Although past data may be adjusted to reflect expected price and other changes, the historical record in the accounting system will provide most of the data for short-range decision analysis. A third difference is the setting of the decisions. Short-range decisions relate to the types, amounts, and prices of services that will be performed with the existing capacity of the organization, while long-range decisions embrace a change in the size of the capacity to provide goods or services.

Nature of Investments

When an organization purchases a long-lived asset, it makes an investment similar to that made by a bank when it lends money. The essential characteristic of both types of transactions is that cash is committed today in the expectation of recovering that cash plus some additional amount in the future. That additional amount is called a *return on investment (ROI)*.

In the case of a bank loan, the ROI is the inflow of interest payments received over the life of the loan. In the case of the long-lived asset, both the return of investment and the return on investment are in the form of cash earnings generated by use of the asset. If, over the life of the investment, the inflows of cash earnings exceed the initial investment outlays (cost), then we know that the original investment was recovered (return of investment) and that some profit was earned (positive ROI). Thus, an investment is the purchase of an expected future stream of cash flows.

When an organization considers whether to purchase a new long-lived asset, the key question is: Will the future cash inflows likely be large enough to justify making the investment? The consideration of these purchases is always framed in the form of a proposal, supported by detailed analysis that contains projections of the streams of expected cash inflows and an evaluation as to whether these inflows will warrant the initial expenditure.

Some of the kinds of proposals typically developed pertain to:

- **Replacement.** Should the organization replace existing equipment with more efficient equipment? The future expected cash inflows would be the cost savings resulting from lower operating costs or the profits from the additional volume produced by the new equipment or both.

- **Expansion.** Should the practice build or otherwise acquire a new facility? The future expected cash inflows on this investment are the cash profits from the goods and services produced in the new facility.

- **Cost reduction.** Should the medical group buy equipment to perform an operation or activity now done manually? That is, should it spend money to save money? The expected future cash inflows are the savings resulting from lower operating costs.

- **Choice of equipment**. Which of several proposed equipment items should be purchased for a given purpose? The choice often depends on which item is expected to provide the largest return on the investment.

- **New product or service.** Should a new product or a new service be added to the existing line? The choice depends on whether the expected future cash inflows from the sale of the product or service are large enough to warrant the investment in equipment, additional working capital, and the costs required to make or develop and introduce the new product or service.

- **Lease or buy**. Having decided that the group needs a building or a new piece of equipment, should it be leased or purchased? The choice in this case depends on whether the investment required to buy the asset will earn an adequate return because of the cash inflows that will result from avoiding the lease payments. In this instance, avoiding a cash outflow is equivalent to receiving a cash inflow.

Traditionally, long-range decisions for medical practices have been made based on medical need. If economic considerations were made at all, simple techniques were usually employed that did not embrace expected future cash inflows or the return on giving up cash today for a larger amount in the future. A long-range decision involves an investment of cash in an asset that yields its return over an extended time period. Included should be a summary of what is expected in the market over the life of the capital item. The accounting measurements of income and historical cost are appropriate for performance evaluation and for providing the relevant information to make short-range decisions. However, because of the long period of time involved in long-range decisions, it is important to consider the time value of money.

Conducting and Communicating Utilization Analyses

Utilization Analysis

Utilization reports present a summary of the various services provided by the group to its patients for a period of time. Three major areas covered by utilization reports pertain to medical services, laboratory testing, and X-ray results. Details of each of these services should be shown, such as patient, type of medical procedures and treatments rendered, responsible physician, type of test, and, if appropriate, applicable costs. The reports may also present year-to-date cumulative totals for each service area and may also be arranged to include previous totals for comparative analysis.

Nonfinancial Measures of Performance

Most performance evaluations focus on financial information taken from the basic accounting data in the financial management system. But, an overall analysis of a medical group's operations should also include nonfinancial information since money only reflects one aspect of resource utilization. The quantitative element not expressed in financial terms has equal importance. Thus, nonfinancial measures should be integrated with a sophisticated financial management system for an overall balanced picture of group operations.

There are different types of nonfinancial performance measures. The easiest to obtain include these aggregates:

- Number of patient visits;
- Number of procedures performed;
- Number of physicians;
- Any changes in physician FTE status
- Number of physician days;
- Number of employees;
- Number of employee workdays;
- Number of hours worked;
- Number of laboratory procedures;
- Number of hospital days; and
- Quantity of supplies used or purchased.

Standing alone, any one of these aggregates is not very useful. However, over time and in combination with other information, they can show important trends that can be compared with historical performance or with data from other groups.

Thus, a more useful type of nonfinancial performance measure combines separate indicators to show various relationships. The most common relationship involves the level of activity and use of resources per FTE physician. Another involves resources used per patient visit or procedure. The following is a list of some of these common indicators:

- Number of scheduled physician office hours;
- Number of various procedures performed;

- Number of missed appointments;
- Number of workdays per physician by specialty;
- Turnover rate or count of termed employees;
- Number of calls completed to patients reminding them of regular checkups;
- Number of patients referred to outside specialists;
- Data related to promoting the practice (e.g., results of using advertisements);
- Monthly average number of prepaid plan members;
- New enrollees (total during quarter);
- Disenrollees (total during quarter);
- Prepaid capitation payment per 1,000 members per month;
- Prepaid charges (FFS equivalent) per 1,000 members per month;
- Outside physician referral expense per 1,000 members per month;
- Outside laboratory referral expense per 1,000 members per month;
- Outside X-ray referral expense per 1,000 members per month;
- Inpatient admissions per 1,000 members per month;
- Payer mix by percentage of charges
- Reimbursement trend line
- Average length of stay per inpatient admission; and
- Physician outpatient encounter per 1,000 members per month.

Forecasting Capital Needs

Determining how much capital a practice needs means the difference between stagnating and growing, and often between thriving and failing. Medical groups need capital for many reasons; the most common reasons are discussed next.

Growing and optimizing the existing practice. For most multispecialty clinics, initiatives that enhance revenues and patient growth are part of their business strategy. None of these types of groups is satisfied with the status quo. Of course, implementing a growth strategy takes capital to hire physicians, build practices, develop new practice locations, contract with health plans, and market to consumers.

The reality is that growth involves an element of risk. The larger the risk in proportion to the operating base of the existing organization, the stronger the argument for outside capital. By outside capital, we are referring to bank loans, leasing, or obtaining funds from hospitals or other sources.

Adding primary care physicians and sites. Primary care network development continues to be one of the more controversial and prevalent and most necessary uses of funds. Large multispecialty groups add locations and build their own primary care bases. The need to acquire primary care practices is often important for multispecialty clinics that use these practices to support insurance contracts that will generate referrals to specialists or to serve health plan subscribers. Many multispecialty clinics have significant primary care networks. Although some sites are built from scratch, many are acquired from physicians with established practices.

Although acquisition of primary care practices may not generate positive direct returns, it is an excellent strategy, especially for multispecialty clinics and integrated healthcare systems. In certain situations, it is also a reasonable strategy for hospitals and health plans. There are ample opportunities to structure primary care investments in such a way that they do not incur significant losses, even on a direct accounting basis.

Investing in new profit centers. Physicians often have the opportunity to invest in new business ventures. These include outpatient surgery centers, provider-owned health plans, medical office buildings, or a piece of medical equipment (e.g., MRI, catheterization lab, etc.). These investments tend to be risky, capital-intensive endeavors. However, for many medical groups, the upside potential more than justifies the risk.

207

The following are examples of situations in which new profit centers might be identified:

- A practice internalizes its diagnostic equipment;
- A group practice and its hospital affiliate jointly develop an ambulatory surgery center; or
- A physician management services organization buys a former hospital and converts it into a diagnostic center.

In the preceding examples, the medical practices required outside capital to meet their strategic goals. Although in many ways disparate, the examples have certain common characteristics:

- The funding requirements and risks are large enough for the medical group to justify a need for outside capital to supplement what it can raise from more conventional sources;
- The upside potential is substantial, more than enough to provide an incentive for outside investors to become involved; and
- The implications for physicians go beyond the new profit centers themselves; the strategic implications often redefine the business purpose of the medical group.

Adding next-generation facilities and equipment. Compared with several of the emerging needs for funding, such as primary care network development and the acquisition of clinical information systems, the need for capital to build new offices and purchase equipment seems mundane. However, it is not. These requirements continue, and with rapid technology advances in medical equipment, there is no easy solution at hand.

In addition to the requisites for modernized and expanded facilities, many clinics need to move to new locations, either adjacent to a hospital or into growth areas. Many hospitals and integrated systems and physician networks are finding that the practices are not in optimal locations for meeting consumer demands. Like banks and supermarkets, the growth of many metropolitan areas is forcing medical groups to move farther out into the suburbs.

With construction costs running well over $250 per square foot for clinic space plus furnishings and equipment, a group of physicians can quickly find themselves in a multimillion dollar building with huge debt service payments.[13]

Adding next-generation information systems. Of all the reasons that medical groups need capital, adding next-generation information systems may be the most important. Every medical group is considering what it needs to do to improve its clinical and management information systems. These systems are essential for contracting managed care, controlling costs, developing clinical guidelines, measuring medical outcomes, and managing the group practice. The development of information systems can be costly but needs to be done. Some of the organizations providing capital for medical groups also offer access to information systems as part of the package.

Developing single-specialty networks. The movement toward medical groups acquiring or merging with other practices has progressed well beyond multispecialty groups. Single-specialty groups are getting together, not only in the same market, but also across markets.

In specialty after specialty — cardiology, neonatology, ophthalmology, oncology, orthopedics, and podiatry — medical practices are exploring opportunities to come together. Their interest in larger single specialty networking is stimulated in part by the chance to invest in new profit centers related to their specialty; however, it is also related to the longer-term potential to provide more coordinated care by focusing on specific diseases and the infrastructure, data, and management systems that would optimize their treatment.

The development of national single-specialty networks, or the acquisition of specialty groups by either multispecialty clinics or other single-specialty clinics also requires significant capital resources. As groups of oncologists, orthopedists, cardiologists, and other specialists consolidate their practices, the accumulation of assets and the costs of clinical and administrative integration often require capital to fund new infrastructure development. In cases involving successful specialists, the capital has tended to be internally generated.

Accepting and managing medical risk. Much of the consolidation of physician practices and their need for capital goes back to the early growth of managed care. Indeed, there appears to be a correlation between the medical groups recognizing that they need capital and the growth of managed care in their markets.

Medical groups must demonstrate the capabilities to perform medical management, such as developing and implementing clinical guidelines and finding transformative ways to deliver care in more cost-effective ways. Developing this infrastructure requires capital.

Covering cash flow shortages. Typical activities within medical group practices include hiring new providers, moving to new offices, adding equipment, and developing new networks. If undertaken by an existing group without adequate capital, they are all likely to lead to short-term reductions in cash flow.

Most medical group administrators work hard to avoid disenchanting their physicians by causing their take-home pay to decline in the pay period after new strategies have been initiated. It has become commonplace in financial transactions to recognize the need for protection against short-term cash flow problems.

Fluctuations in cash flow are very much a part of doing business as a medical group. When special expenses are added on top of the normal cash flow ups and downs, the probabilities of an occasional monthly shortfall increase dramatically. Making sure that the medical group has an adequate base of working capital (usually short-term lines of credit from commercial banks) is one way to guard against these circumstances. *Insulating against risk.* Many healthcare organizations, including hospitals and medical groups, long for the deep pockets of a financial partner. Part of this is in response to the financial resources of several large health plans; hospital systems (both for profit and not for profit); and public and private investors.

There is a sense of security about the future when physicians have access to capital, and this is contributing to physician practices seeking capital partners.

Capital Sources: The Alternatives

As with any business, medical groups have financing sources such as retained earnings, borrowing, and leasing available to them. However, medical groups now have several additional alternatives that are not available to other businesses. These include selling all or a portion of the practice or entering into some other kind of arrangement with a hospital. They can also think about partnering with a health plan.

Here are the six broad options available to medical groups for accessing capital:

1. Retained earnings;

2. Borrowing, usually from a commercial bank or other financial institution;

3. Leasing;

4. Hospitals and multi-hospital systems;

5. Integrated healthcare systems; and

6. Health plans.

Conducting a Financial Analysis

It is important for physicians and management at a medical practice to have a grasp of basic financial statements and analysis tools so they can make sense of the group's finances. These skills can also help root out and even head off trouble if an incompetent or unscrupulous employee or outside consultant is mishandling the company's finances or worse. For an overview of the basic financial statements (balance sheet, income statement, statement of changes in equity, and statement of cash flows), refer to Chapter 3 (pages 115–122).

Exhibit 5.17

Internal Comparisons of Income Statement Data for Current vs. Prior Year

Blue Mountain Orthopedic Group, P.C.
Internal Comparisons of Income Statement Data
For the Years Ended 2015 vs. 2014

	2015	%	2014	%	Net Change	%
Revenues:						
Net fee-for-service revenue	$6,930,000	99.21%	$6,275,000	99.21%	$655,000	10.44%
Capitation Revenue	–	0.00%	–	0.00%	–	
Other	55,000	0.79%	50,000	0.79%	5,000	10.00%
Net Revenue	6,985,000	100.00%	6,325,000	100.00%	660,000	10.43%
Operating Expenses:						
Salary and Fringe Benefits:						
Staff salaries	1,200,000	17.18%	1,100,000	17.39%	100,000	9.09%
Payroll taxes	100,000	1.43%	90,000	1.42%	10,000	11.11%
Employee benefits	300,000	4.29%	250,000	3.95%	50,000	20.00%
Total salary and fringe benefits	1,600,000	22.91%	1,440,000	22.77%	160,000	11.11%
Services and General Expenses						
Malpractice insurance	170,000	2.43%	145,000	2.29%	25,000	17.24%
Provision for bad debts	180,000	2.58%	175,000	2.77%	5,000	2.86%
Medical and surgical supplies	178,000	2.55%	162,000	2.56%	16,000	9.88%
Depreciation	75,000	1.07%	70,000	1.11%	5,000	7.14%
Rent	400,000	5.73%	375,000	5.93%	25,000	6.67%
Information technology	100,000	1.43%	95,000	1.50%	5,000	5.26%
Other general and administrative	388,000	5.55%	367,000	5.80%	21,000	5.72%
Total services and general expense	1,491,000	21.35%	1,389,000	21.96%	102,000	7.34%
Total operating expenses	3,091,000	44.25%	2,829,000	44.73%	262,000	9.26%
Net revenue after operating expenses	3,894,000	55.75%	3,496,000	55.27%	398,000	11.38%
Provider-related expenses:						
Physician salaries and benefits	3,750,000	53.69%	3,370,000	53.28%	380,000	11.28%
Net income after provider-related expense	144,000	2.06%	126,000	1.99%	18,000	14.29%
Other Income (Expense):						
Interest expense (net)	(12,000)	-0.17%	(8,000)	-0.13%	(4,000)	50.00%
Net income before income taxes	132,000	1.89%	118,000	1.87%	14,000	11.86%
Provision for income taxes	45,000	0.64%	42,000	0.66%	3,000	7.14%
Net income	87,000	1.25%	76,000	1.20%	11,000	14.47%
Retained Earnings, Beginning of Year	558,000	7.99%	482,000	7.62%	76,000	15.77%
Retained Earnings, End of Year	$645,000	9.23%	$558,000	8.82%	$87,000	15.59%

Analytical Procedures

Consultants and outside accountants generate many of their suggestions for clients on how to improve their business operations by applying analytical procedures to financial data. Administrators can use the same procedures to determine operational improvements necessary to improve their practices' performance. Examples of analytical procedures include:

- Internal comparisons;
- Ratio analysis; and
- Benchmarking financial data against industry data.

Internal Comparisons

One good way to begin a financial analysis is by reviewing and comparing the practice's internal data. Useful comparisons include:

- Current data vs. prior period data;
- Current actual data vs. budgets, forecasts, or other prospective data; and
- By business segment, such as department, location, or specialty.

Current data vs. prior period data. One popular analysis method is to compare current-year amounts against equivalent prior-year amounts, including variances in terms of both the dollar amount and as a percentage of the prior period balance, and investigating significant variances. This analysis is usually more meaningful when performed on income-statement rather than balance-sheet amounts. Generally, income statement numbers are more stable because they represent a fixed time period, whereas the balance sheet shows amounts at a point in time. Exhibit 5.17 shows this comparison for the fictitious medical practice first introduced in Chapter 3, Blue Mountain Orthopedic Group, P.C.

Some popular accounting packages have report-writer modules that can generate this report. Outside accountants who prepare practice financial statements may also be able to generate these reports through their client accounting software.

Current actual data vs. budgets, forecasts, or other prospective data. Practice administrators can use the same format as that shown in Exhibit 5.17 to compute differences between the current period actual numbers and those contained in budgets, forecasts, or other prospective analyses.

By business segment. Comparing financial data among business segments such as practice locations, specialties, or other divisions is a useful technique for discovering inefficiencies, underperformers, best practices, and accounting errors. These comparisons can be done using actual amounts, but they are often more meaningful when comparing ratios.

Financial Benchmarking

Webster's New Collegiate Dictionary defines *benchmarking* as "a standard by which something can be measured or judged."[14] The Xerox Corporation says that benchmarking is "the continuous process of measuring products, services, and practices against the toughest competitors or those companies recognized as industry leaders (best in class)."[15]

Our society benchmarks many activities, ranging from business and industry to leisure pursuits. Automobile manufacturers benchmark miles per gallon and annual fuel costs because that data must be displayed on new car window stickers. Major appliance manufacturers must post energy efficiency ratings on all appliances to compare energy usage against similar appliances. Sports benchmarks include batting averages for baseball players and efficiency ratings for football quarterbacks.

Benchmarking has come to healthcare in reports of top hospitals, managed care premium networks, and, more recently, pay for performance.

For medical practices, benchmarking is another financial analysis tool for improving performance. Medical groups can apply the benchmarking process both internally and externally to identify opportunities for operational improvement.

The major benefits of benchmarking are that it lets a medical practice:

- Measure its performance;
- Quantify its performance relative to others;
- Identify opportunities for improvement;
- Generate new ideas and creative thinking;
- Provide a basis for strategic planning;
- Use an objective, data-driven process that is generally accepted by physicians; and
- Encourage teamwork and collaboration.
- Trend line for future forecasting
- Benchmarking does have limitations, including:
- One benchmark is not enough;
- The numbers tell one piece of the overall story
- Practices must benchmark results and processes;
- Benchmarking requires time and thought;
- Comparison data are never perfect;
- Comparison data may not be timely;
- Benchmarking requires open, honest, and objective assessments; and
- It requires the mutual sharing of benchmarking information.

MGMA provides external benchmarking information to medical practices through many of its products and services. Its annual cost and physician compensation and production surveys and its *Data Dive™ Modules* and *Performances and Practices of Successful Medical Groups* provide comparative statistical data regarding medical practice performance. Many other organizations also provide relevant external benchmarking information, including the American Medical Association, the American Medical Group Association, the Association of American Medical Colleges, and a number of physician specialty societies.

Before attempting to create benchmarks, it is important to understand the benchmarking process. A practice must be selective about what it attempts to benchmark, and it must benchmark those areas that can be changed by management. The customary steps in the benchmarking process are:

1. Identify the areas of the practice to be reviewed and improved;

2. Understand the practice's current process or information;

3. Determine specific processes or results to be benchmarked;

4. Identify peer groups and source information;

5. Collect and compile accurate data;

6. Analyze results;

7. Make recommendations for improvement;

8. Implement recommendations; and

9. Measure and report the results.

10. Develop plans and take action as needed

Most medical practices benchmark data internally, externally, or both. Internal benchmarking includes physician to physician, office to office, and service line to service line.

In external benchmarking, the practice compares physician productivity and clinical quality to external clinical benchmarks and financial results to external benchmarks in business areas. Exhibits 5.18 through 5.21 are examples of benchmarking for the fictitious practice Deep South Obstetrics and Gynecology, P.C. (any resemblance to an actual practice is purely coincidental).[16]

A careful review of areas in which the practice is significantly over or under the benchmark will identify areas that are functioning very well and those that need improvement. This also allows a practice to establish and manage a continuous improvement mindset.

Presenting Financial Results to Stakeholders

Although the administrator frequently performs much of the practice's financial analysis, physicians and other stakeholders often have the ultimate responsibility for practice activities and major financial decisions. For example, the governing body anticipates cash flow and assesses management's performance. It makes crucial decisions on whether to add another physician, buy a building, offer ancillary services, and many other issues.

To fulfill these responsibilities, decision makers need timely and relevant information on the practice's financial performance. On some occasions, they may need special analyses such as an ROI or cost-benefit the administrator must ensure that these stakeholders not only receive this information, but that they understand it well enough to make informed decisions. This task can be especially challenging when some decision makers have limited financial knowledge. At the same time, however, the administrator must present enough financial detail to those stakeholders who are financially astute.

Providing Information

The administrator should provide agreed-upon financial reports to physicians and other stakeholders on a regular basis. These normally include financial statements, budget comparisons, billing information, and clinical productivity metrics. Depending on the nature of the practice, stakeholders may want other reports, such as incoming/ outgoing referrals, cancellations and no-shows, or appointment availability. Providing a dashboard of summary financial data gives an executive summary of practice performance.

Some of the most important reporting projects are those special reports that the administrator prepares on an as-needed basis to facilitate a particular decision, such as whether to invest in an electronic health record system or whether to change the way the group's employee health insurance is handled.

Exhibit 5.18
Benchmark against MGMA Cost Survey Overall per FTE Physician[17]

DEEP SOUTH OBSTETRICS AND GYNECOLOGY, P.C.

		2013			
	Practice $	Practice $ per FTE Physician	MGMA Cost Benchmark	Practice over (under) MGMA Benchmark $	%
Revenues:					
Net fee-for-service revenue	$5,600,000	$800,000	$807,429	($7,429)	−1%
Operation Expenses					
Salaries and benefits:					
Support staff salaries	$1,246,000	$178,000	$156,916	$21,084	13%
Employee benefits and taxes	$295,001	$42,143	$42,714	($571)	−1%
Total salaries and benefits (sum of above)	$1,541,001	$220,143	$199,630	$20,513	10%
Total salaries and benefits (from survey)			$191,718	$28,425	15%
Services and general expenses:					
Information technology	$140,000	$20,000	$18,410	$1,590	9%
Drug supply	$108,500	$15,500	$14,683	$817	6%
Medical and surgical supply	$315,000	$45,000	$41,299	$3,701	9%
Building and occupancy	$330,001	$47,143	$48,336	($1,193)	−2%
Furniture and equipment	$28,000	$4,000	$3,662	$338	9%
Furniture/equipment depreciation	$28,000	$4,000	$4,484	($484)	−11%
Admin supplies and services	$70,000	$10,000	$9,863	$137	1%
Professional liability insurance	$217,000	$31,000	$28,004	$2,996	11%
Other insurance premiums	$10,500	$1,500	$1,423	$77	5%
Legal fees	$10,500	$1,500	$1,426	$74	5%
Outside professional fees	$28,000	$4,000	$4,590	($590)	−13%
Promotion and marketing	$26,005	$3,715	$4,215	($500)	−12%
Miscellaneous operating cost	$70,000	$10,000	$9,237	$763	8%
Total general operating cost (from sum of above)	$1,381,506	$197,358	$189,632	$7,726	4%
Total general operating cost (from cost survey)			$237,527	($40,169)	−17%

DEEP SOUTH OBSTETRICS AND GYNECOLOGY, P.C.

| | | 2013 | | | |
| | | Practice $ per FTE Physician | MGMA Cost Benchmark | Practice over (under) MGMA Benchmark | |
	Practice $			$	%
Provider-related expenses:					
Physician salaries	$1,995,000	$285,000	$294,185	($9,185)	−3%
Physician benefits and taxes	$217,000	$31,000	$26,017	$4,983	19%
Total physician costs from (sum of above)	$2,212,000	$316,000			
Total physician costs (from survey)			$311,529	$4,471	1%
Nonphysician provider salaries	$350,000	$50,000	$52,505	($2,505)	−5%
Nonphysician provider benefits and taxes	$63,000	$9,000	$8,811	$189	2%
Total nonphysician provider costs (sum of above)	$413,000	$59,000			
Total nonphysician provider costs (from survey)			$52,890	$6,110	12%
Total provider costs (sum of above)	$2,625,000	$375,000			
Total provider costs (from survey)			$359,052		
Total cost (from survey)	$5,547,507	$792,501	$781,465		
Income from operations	$52,493	$7,499			
Income (Loss) (from survey)			$4,680		
FTE physicians	7				
FTE nonphysician providers	3				

Exhibit 5.19

Benchmark against MGMA Cost Survey Overall Percentage of Total Medical Revenue[18]

DEEP SOUTH OBSTETRICS AND GYNECOLOGY, P.C.

			2013	
	Practice		MGMA	Practice over (under) MGMA Benchmark
	$	%	Benchmark	%
Revenues:				
Net fee-for-service revenue	$5,600,000	100%	100.00%	
Salaries and benefits:				
Staff salaries	$1,246,000	22%	19.41%	3%
Employee benefits and taxes	$295,001	5%	5.87%	−1%
Total salaries and benefits (from survey)	1,541,001	28%	24.14%	3%
Services and general expenses:				
Information technology	$140,000	3%	2.07%	0%
Drug supply	$108,500	2%	1.52%	0%
Medical and surgical supply	$315,000	6%	4.65%	1%
Building and occupancy	$330,001	6%	6.28%	0%
Furniture and equipment	$28,000	1%	—	1%
Furniture/equipment depreciation	$28,000	1%	0.39%	0%
Admin supplies and services	$70,000	1%	0.52%	1%
Professional liability insurance	$217,000	4%	1.42%	2%
Other insurance premiums	$10,500	0%	3.24%	−3%
Legal fees	$10,500	0%	0.24%	0%
Outside professional fees	$28,000	1%	0.15%	0%
Promotion and marketing	$26,005	0%	—	0%
Miscellaneous operating cost	$70,000	1%	0.66%	1%
Total general operating cost (from sum of above)	$1,381,506	25%	0.57%	24%
Total general operating cost (from survey)			29.77%	−30%

DEEP SOUTH OBSTETRICS AND GYNECOLOGY, P.C.

	Practice $	Practice %	MGMA Benchmark	Practice over (under) MGMA Benchmark %
2013				
Provider-related expenses:	$1,995,000	36%		36%
Physician salaries	$217,000	4%	34.61%	−31%
Physician benefits and taxes	$2,212,000	40%	2.71%	37%
Total physician costs (from survey)			36.38%	−36%
Nonphysician provider salaries	$350,000	6%	5.15%	1%
Nonphysician provider benefits and taxes	$63,000	1%	0.76%	0%
Total nonphysician provider costs (from survey)	$413,000	7%	5.48%	2%
Total provider costs (from sum of above)	$2,625,000	47%		
Total provider costs (from survey)			39.10%	
Total cost (from survey)	$5,547,507	99%	100.25%	
Nonmedical costs				
Interest and taxes				
Income (Loss)	$52,493	1%	0.37%	

Exhibit 5.20
Benchmark against MGMA Cost Survey Staffing per FTE Physician[19]

DEEP SOUTH OBSTETRICS AND GYNECOLOGY, P.C.

	FTE Practice	FTE per FTE Physician	2013 MGMA Cost Benchmark	Practice over (under) MGMA Benchmark FTE	%
Business operations support staff					
General administrative	2.00	0.29	0.33	(0.04)	−13%
Patient accounting	4.00	0.57	0.60	(0.03)	−5%
Total business operations support staff	7.00	1.00	1.07	(0.07)	−7%
Total front office support staff	11.00	1.57	1.33	0.24	18%
Clinical support staff					
Registered nurses	4.00	0.57	0.47	0.10	22%
Licensed practical nurses	3.00	0.43	0.55	(0.12)	−22%
Medical assistants, nurses aides	6.00	0.86	0.94	(0.08)	−9%
Total clinical support	13.00	1.86	1.78	0.08	4%
Ancillary support staff					
Clinical laboratory	1.50	0.21	—	0.21	
Radiology and imaging	3.50	0.50	0.43	0.07	16%
Total ancillary support staff	5.00	0.71	0.38	0.33	88%
Total support staff (sum of above)	35.00	5.00			
Total support staff (from survey)			4.85	0.15	3%
Total FTE physicians	7.00		5.13		
Total FTE nonphysician providers	3.00		3.8		

Explaining Financial Information

Whereas financially astute administrators may take pride in their detailed financial analyses, these analyses may confuse some stakeholders. This section discusses tools and techniques that administrators have used successfully to communicate financial information to their governing bodies. The success of a particular method will vary depending on the attributes of the situation, the practice, the administrator, and the individual stakeholders.

Using Words to Explain Numbers

Administrators have reported success using both written and oral communication to explain financial data to stakeholders, such as letters, group presentations, and one-on-one discussions.

Letters, memos, and executive summaries from management. Providing a management letter with the regular financial reports offers an interpretation of the numbers and insight into what is happening in the practice. Consider the following example:

> As you can see, the total charges and the number of procedures are up for the year-to-date compared to last year. These increases are primarily a result of increased patient volume at the East Side Clinic.

> Unfortunately, collections for August were lower than expected. This occurred because we had difficulty getting paid by ABC Healthcare. Evidently this payer's recent computer update resulted in a "bug" in its system that mistakenly rejected our claims as noncovered services. ABC was able to fix the bug, and we received these payments in early September.

Memos and executive summaries are one or two pages in length and include all the sections of a typical document in short form. Memos tend to be less formal and loosely formatted, whereas executive summaries should adhere to the structure of a formal report, containing:[21]

- From, To, Subject, Body, Salutation, Signature;
- Introduction, Background, Definitions, Problem Statement, Procedure, Results, Examples, Discussion; and,
- Statement of purpose and rationale, theoretical framework, research questions, key terms and variables, definition of population of interest, description of research design, assumptions and limitations, implications of findings, dissemination of findings.

Exhibit 5.21

Benchmark against MGMA with Compensation[20]

DEEP SOUTH OBSTETRICS AND GYNECOLOGY, P.C.

Physician/Extender	Days Off	Practice Type	Professional Charges	Collections
Smith	45	GYN	650,000	300,000
% of Benchmark	129%		93%	92%
Jones	40	GYN	800,000	425,000
% of Benchmark	114%		115%	130%
MGMA Median	35		696,255	327,192
Harris	32	OB/GYN	1,200,000	600,000
% of Benchmark	91%		137%	115%
Thruman	30	OB/GYN	1,300,000	675,000
% of Benchmark	86%		148%	129%
Dunn	20	OB/GYN	1,500,000	750,000
% of Benchmark	57%		171%	144%
Thompson	25	OB/GYN	1,200,000	600,000
% of Benchmark	71%		137%	115%
Cohen	30	OB/GYN	1,200,000	650,000
% of Benchmark	86%		137%	125%
MGMA Median	35		877,845	521,418
Nurse Practitioner				
Bence	20	Office	225,000	175,000
% of Benchmark			99%	115%
Davis	25	Office	200,000	155,000
% of Benchmark			88%	102%
MGMA Median			227,188	152,215
Starr	25	Hospital		
Total Nurse Practitioner			227,188	152,215

	Encounters			Hospital			Total
Office	Hospital	Total	Cases	Ultrasounds	RVUs	Comp.
2,000	75	2,075	125	275	7,500	225,000
87%	99%	87%	93%	0%	86%	140%
2,400	115	2,515	175	325	9,000	225,000
104%	151%	106%	130%	0%	103%	140%
2,298	76	2,374	135	–	8,724	160,510
3,100	140	3,240	310	350	12,000	270,000
103%	100%	103%	94%	0%	103%	115%
3,500	155	3,655	325	375	12,500	280,000
116%	111%	116%	99%	0%	107%	119%
3,750	210	3,960	375	425	13,750	325,000
124%	150%	125%	114%	0%	118%	138%
3,100	135	3,235	300	325	12,000	265,000
103%	96%	103%	91%	0%	103%	113%
3,050	150	3,200	315	350	12,300	275,000
101%	107%	101%	96%	0%	105%	117%
3,016	140	3,156	329	–	11,661	235,000
2,200					6,000	65,000
137%					125%	104%
2,400					5,500	65,000
149%					114%	104%
1,607					4,818	62,789
						66,000
1,607	–	–	–	–	4,818	196,000

General correspondence and e-mails should follow the KISS (keep it short and simple) principle. For example, if there were multiple important issues that needed to be addressed by the physician staff, in keeping with the KISS principle, only one topic should be addressed in detail per e-mail or correspondence. That is, they should be one page in length and cover one topic. General correspondence and e-mails should be used to relay a single thought, piece of information, or topic using the least number of words with few graphs or charts. In addition, the writing should be professional and adhere to accepted methods of grammar, punctuation, and spelling. In particular, the writing style in e-mails has evolved into a unique use of acronyms and symbols (e.g., LOL for laugh out loud or smiley faces using a combination of keys) and these acronyms and symbols should be used sparingly for emphasis.

Because e-mails are easily shared (forwarded), the importance of maintaining professionalism cannot be understated — how you are perceived will be decided by your e-mail style. A poor first impression can easily result from a poorly crafted e-mail message. Furthermore, the use of e-mail requires discretion and patience because of its capabilities and speed of delivery. Because most e-mails are short, sending a lengthy narrative with multiple attachments will quickly prompt a receiver to hit "delete." And an e-mail sent in haste or in the heat of the moment can easily snowball into a serious problem you might regret (e.g., sending an emotional e-mail with excessive exclamation marks and four-letter words to your boss). Also, unlike any other method of communication, aside from verbal, once the e-mail has been sent, the opportunity to proofread or edit has passed.

Oral presentations. The administrator will often have to explain financial information at board meetings. Good presentation skills, including the ability to discuss complex financial matters in common terms, are essential.

When giving presentations, consider the following guidelines:

- Limit your presentation to less than one hour (provide at least 10 minutes for questions and answers); if you tell your audience the presentation will be 50 minutes, stick to your 50 minutes;

- Identify your audience and design around your audience (What are your audience's expectations, background, education, etc.?);
- Determine the purpose of your presentation;
- Ensure that the text font is consistent throughout and large enough to be seen from a distance
- Limit the number of characters per slide (too much text is distracting and difficult to see use of bullet points is highly effective
- Special effects should be used sparingly (using animation, action settings, and sound can be distracting);
- Images should be used in moderation but can be used to consume white space (real-life pictures are preferable to clip art);
- Limit the total number of slides based on other considerations (How much time do you have and how long does it take to present a slide?);
- Structure the presentation logically (title, outline or agenda, content, summary, question and answer);
- Maintain professionalism, dress properly, and do not use slang or technical jargon;
- Move around (try not to stand in one place like a statue);
- Use your hands to talk in a mature manner, but remember this is not a karate demonstration so don't get carried away;
- Plan, prepare, and take a break from your presentation, then reread and reproof;
- Arrive early to the presentation room (walk around the room to get comfortable with it and check to make sure equipment works and the presentation can be read from the back of the room);
- Do not read from your presentation; use it to supplement, illustrate, and organize;
- Answer questions honestly and respectfully; and
- Adequate preparation is essential.

One-on-one discussions. These can be useful with stakeholders of all levels of financial knowledge. The administrator can explain financial basics to those without financial backgrounds. This gives stakeholders who are not experts an opportunity to ask questions privately, which is something they may be hesitant to do in a larger group.

For financially astute shareholders, one-on-one discussions can provide a venue for in-depth discussions of financial issues, complete with technical language. Physicians with the stronger financial backgrounds can often help explain these issues to other physicians.

Bars and Graphs

Seeing is believing. Converting technical financial data to pie charts, graphs, and bar charts creates something all members of the group can understand. Inserting one or more of these graphics into a memo or management report makes the message clearer. Each visual should be used with a clear purpose in mind. For example, to present:[22]

- Frequencies of discrete data, use a bar chart;
- Frequencies of continuous data, use a histogram;
- Percentages (relative frequencies), use a pie chart;
- Trends of continuous data, use a line graph, and;
- Relationships between two variables, use a scatter plot.

No matter the type of graph, it should always indicate which direction you want to the data to be headed.

Dashboards and Other Technology

Dashboards are typically visual representations of metrics, benchmarks, practice activities, and process status in a single (or few) display screens. For example, a relative value unit (RVU) dashboard might show physician work RVUs by physician in a line graph with an exhibit populated by the attached number of RVUs. In addition, the line graph might contain a line representing the practice average and a line depicting the MGMA average for the practice's specialty. In addition, a dashboard has multiple layers for displaying different practice metrics; when the cursor is placed over chart areas, additional information is automatically displayed.

Ultimately, a dashboard functions as a one-stop shop for quickly monitoring, comparing, and identifying current status and potential problems, serving as an excellent early warning tool. Dashboards improve management capabilities by automating data collection, display, and analysis. They also eliminate tedious hours of number crunching and analysis, and speed decision response time driven by readily available, real-time practice information.

Many practices have automated dashboards that use internet, corporate intranet, and database technologies. This enables users to access the dashboard from any computer with internet connectivity. In addition, the benefits of web-enabling a dashboard permits custom calculations, flexibility, and real-time availability of practice measures.

Today's technology provides options beyond the paper report for distributing financial information. Administrators can e-mail the files or put the information on a CD or DVD. A web portal can provide online access to prepared reports or real-time access to financial data. These portals allow stakeholders to select the amount of detail they wish to view. Some may review the dashboard and various bars and graphs, whereas others may study the detailed data in the supporting spreadsheets.

Ultimately, dashboards and reports are only useful if they result in action or decision-making. Administrators can be overwhelmed by the amount of data available to them, so focusing their attention on those indicators that drive successful performance of strategic objectives is crucial. To deliver results, action plans with specific timelines and assigned to those responsible must be developed and monitored. Always remember that a goal without a plan is just a wish.

Conclusion

Budgeting is a multifaceted exercise that affects medical practices on a daily basis. The effective practice administrator should have knowledge of accounting systems, budget methodologies, and elements of financial statements, and skill in financial forecasting, developing budgets, investment management, financial analysis, and benchmarking and communicating financial results to key stakeholders.

Notes

1. These sample financial statements were adapted from the online course materials for *Financial Management Boot Camp: Self-Study* (Englewood, CO: Medical Group Management Association, 2014), www.mgma.com/store/education/online/ courses-self-study/ financial-management-boot-camp-self-study.

2. Charles T. Horngren, Srikant M. Datar, and George Foster, *Cost Accounting: A Managerial Emphasis* (Upper Saddle River, NJ: Prentice Hall, 2002), 193.

3. Greg Brue and Rod Howes, *The McGraw-Hill 36-Hour Course: Six Sigma* (New York: McGraw-Hill, 2006), 59.

4. Horngren et al., *Cost Accounting*, 178.

5. *Publication 946: How to Depreciate Property* (Cat. No. 13081F), Internal Revenue Service, Feb. 27, 2015, http://www.irs.gov/pub/irs-pdf/p946.pdf.

6. *Publication 946*.

7. Horngren et al., *Cost Accounting*, 3.

8. Horngren et al., *Cost Accounting*.

9. This example was adapted from Frederic R. Simmons and Lee Ann H. Webster, "Cost Management and Cost Accounting in the Medical Practice" (MGMA Preconference Program, Las Vegas, NV, Oct. 22, 2006).

10. Horngren et al., *Cost Accounting*, 836.

11. Horngren et al., *Cost Accounting*, 837.

12. Horngren et al., *Cost Accounting*, 31.

13. *Financial Management for Medical Groups: A Resource for New and Experienced Managers*, 3rd ed. (Englewood, CO: MGMA, 2014), 506.

14. *Webster's New Collegiate Dictionary*, 150th anniversary ed., s.v. "benchmarking."

15. David T. Kearns, "Quality Improvement Begins at the Top," *World 20*, 21, no. 5 (May 1986).

16. These examples were adapted from Simmons and Webster, "Cost Management and Cost Accounting in the Medical Practice."

17. MGMA Cost Benchmark from *MGMA Cost Survey: 2014 Report Based on 2013 Data*.

18. MGMA Cost Benchmark from *MGMA Cost Survey: 2014 Report Based on 2013 Data*.

19. MGMA Cost Benchmark from *MGMA Cost Survey: 2014 Report Based on 2013 Data*.

20. MGMA Benchmark from *MGMA Physician Compensation and Production Survey, 2004 Report Based on 2003 Data*, Tables 23, 43, 50, 52, 54 and 2.

21. D. Lynn Kelley, *Measurement Made Accessible: A Research Approach Using Qualitative, Quantitative, and Quality Improvement Methods* (Thousand Oaks, CA: Sage, 1999); S. Plichta (Old Dominion University, Norfolk, VA), personal communications, 2001–2005.

22. Kelley, *Measurement Made Accessible*; Plichta, personal communications.

Chapter 6

Audits and Internal Controls

Auditing is the systematic process of objectively obtaining and evaluating the accounts or financial records of a business entity based on established criteria. While auditing focuses largely on financial information, the process may also involve the inspection or examination of a particular business process to evaluate or improve its appropriateness, safety, or efficiency and reporting the results to key stakeholders. Key skills required to manage the auditing process include understanding the types of audits, establishing internal audit processes, identifying when external audits are necessary, complying with accepted auditing standards, and identifying opportunities to improve operations based on audit results.

Types of Audits

There are three main types of audits: financial statement audits, operational audits, and compliance audits.

Financial Statement Audit

The independent examination of an organization's financial statements is called a financial statement audit. The audit report provided in this setting gives assurance to external users that the financial statements are prepared in accordance with established criteria, such as generally accepted accounting principles (GAAP). There are other types of audit activities that can be performed, which provide benefits to the organization.

Operational Audit

An operational audit is performed to determine the extent to which some aspect of an organization's operating activities is functioning effectively and efficiently. In these audits, auditors observe and test various areas of one or more of a firm's activities, such as the production process of a manufacturing company. Operational audits would assess the performance of the production process, identify opportunities for improving the process, and develop recommendations for upgrading company activities. Unlike a financial statement audit, the reports and analyses generated by an operational audit would not circulate externally but would be used by management only.

Compliance Audit

A compliance audit is conducted to determine the extent to which an organization and/or its personnel are performing their duties in a manner consistent with organizational policies and procedures. For example, a common organizational policy relates to the adherence to internal control procedures. Such a compliance audit would be conducted to identify deviations from these procedures.

Another type of compliance audit would deal with an organization's compliance with federal laws, regulations, contracts, and grants. For example, an audit might be performed to investigate whether funds received from various sources were used for the specified purposes. In medical practices, there might be a compliance audit to tell whether the accounting procedures for billing patients were in compliance with Medicare and Medicaid regulations. Another example is coding audits whereby internal or external coding experts will exam a random sample of documentation assuring their compliance to acceptable coding rules. The results of the audit should be reported to key stakeholders and reviewed with the providers in a timely manner for corrective action planning if necessary.

There are also tax compliance audits performed by the Internal Revenue Service (IRS) and state tax agents.

234

Financial Audits

Accounting is a process of collecting, summarizing, and communicating financial information about economic events and their results as they relate to business entities. There are various groups besides the owners who have an interest in the economic affairs of these entities. For public corporations, these groups might be investors, creditors, financial analysts, governmental officials, employees, and others concerned with the operations of the business. For medical practices, these external parties might be creditors, suppliers, third-party reimbursement entities, and other governmental agencies.

Among these parties, there is a need for assurance that the financial statements prepared and distributed by management contain information that is fairly presented in accordance with GAAP. The purpose of auditing is to provide an independent process that ensures that the statements can be relied on to depict what they purport to represent. There are four key aspects of the auditing process that help to add to the credibility of the financial statements:

1. Auditing is a systematic process based on logic and reasoning. It is planned and conducted in a methodical, not haphazard, manner.

2. The auditor obtains and evaluates evidence. Evidence is collected throughout the audit as the auditor makes decisions about the financial information presented by management's financial statements.

3. The evidence compiled by the auditor is used to ascertain the degree of correspondence between the assertions (elements on the financial statements prepared by management) and established criteria (GAAP).

4. Finally, the auditor communicates the results of the audit to interested parties, such as stockholders, creditors, and so on. The communication is called the *auditor's report.*

Independent auditors (usually certified public accountants, or CPAs) conduct audits and render an opinion in their audit reports about the fairness of the presentation of financial statements issued by management. This process is called *attestation*, and an audit is sometimes referred to as an *attest engagement*.

Coding Audits

The complexity of coding and documenting professional services makes it likely that providers may at times miscode services at a higher or lower level than what is considered proper or fail to provide enough documentation to justify the code selected. *Downcoding*, which is entering a lower-than-appropriate code, causes lower reimbursements and skews measurements of provider productivity. Coding at a higher-than-justified level, that is, upcoding, can lead payers to suspect fraud. The repercussions can include payer audits of the practice's records, or worse, civil or criminal charges against the provider and possible suspension or exclusion from the payer's program. Therefore, it is critical that administrators implement a program of compliance with federal billing and coding requirements. The Office of Inspector General for Health and Human Services, which has the authority to exclude providers from the Medicare and Medicaid programs, recommends that a practice routinely review bills and medical notes for compliance with coding, billing, and documentation requirements.

When initiating a compliance program, the practice must determine whether to review claims retrospectively or concurrently as they are submitted.[1] The auditing system can begin with a baseline audit, only examining claims submitted during the three-month period immediately after the compliance program begins. Follow-up audits should be conducted at least annually to ensure that the practice's compliance program is being followed. For newer providers, training for proper coding and the oversight process should be part of their on-boarding activities. They should continue receive a higher number of audits until results of audits are consistent, safeguarding from long-term coding compliance issues. At a minimum, the practice should review the claims it has submitted for reimbursement from federal programs. One of the most important components of an audit protocol is making an appropriate response when a problem is detected. This may include refunding overpayments to payers, implementing compliance standards, increasing provider education, and, in cases of deliberate miscoding, enforcing disciplinary actions. It also advisable that refunds or repayments to federal, state or commercial payers be addressed in the compensation methodology section of employment agreements with providers.

Revenue Audits

Practices need to devote sufficient resources to ensure that the amounts of net revenue (fee-for-service revenue, capitation revenue, pay for performance and any other revenues) in the financial statements are a reasonably accurate representation of the amounts the practice will ultimately collect.[2] Incorrectly computing these amounts leads to a misleading financial statement that can overstate or understate the revenues on which physicians' bonuses or other compensation is computed. It may also cause the practice to run short of cash, miss instances of underpayment by payers and mistakes by outsourced billing companies, and, potentially, to negotiate less-than-favorable fees in future contracts with insurance companies. Discovery of errors relating to revenue audits need to be reported immediately and verified to ensure that the issue has been addressed and proper controls are in place.

The Audit Report

Audit examinations are carried out following a prescribed set of standards that measure the quality of the auditor's performance as well as the objectives to be attained by using certain procedures. These auditing standards rarely change, and if they do, it's only because of the official decree of the Auditing Standards Board, a professional body of CPAs who constantly monitor the effectiveness of existing standards and developments. Generally accepted auditing standards (GAAS) are important for several reasons:

- To define the broad objectives of every independent audit;

- To provide a gauge for judging an auditor's performance; and

- To set recognized standards of the profession through the business and legal world.

There are ten GAAS, which are divided into three broad categories: (1) general standards, (2) standards of fieldwork, and (3) standards of reporting. These standards, as developed by the Auditing Standards Board and approved by the members of the American Institute of Certified Public Accountants (AICPA; the professional organization of CPAs), are listed in Exhibit 6.1. Financial managers should be aware of these standards when they assess their practice's internal and external auditing services.

Auditors' reports are addressed to the governing body of the organization requesting the audit. An introductory paragraph identifies the responsibilities of both the client (e.g., XYZ Company) and the auditor regarding the financial statements. The second paragraph contains the auditor's description of the scope of the examination and is called the *scope paragraph*. In the third paragraph, the auditor renders an opinion about the fairness of the presentation of the financial statements in what is usually referred to as the *opinion paragraph*. The report is signed by a partner of the CPA firm involved. The date printed on the report is the actual date the audit fieldwork was completed. This indicates the point at which the auditor was in a position to render an opinion.

An unqualified audit opinion, illustrated in Exhibit 6.2, means that the auditor believes that the financial statements are presented fairly, that they conform with GAAP, that they are applied consistently each year, and that the statements include all necessary disclosures. It means that the statements fairly present the financial position, results of operations, and cash flows.

Besides the unqualified opinion, auditors can render three other types of opinions:

1. A *qualified opinion* in which the auditor expresses certain reservations in the report regarding the scope

Exhibit 6.1
Generally Accepted Auditing Standards[3]

General Standards

1. The auditor must have adequate technical training and proficiency to perform the audit.

2. The auditor must maintain independence in mental attitude in all matters relating to the audit.

3. The auditor must exercise due professional care in the performance of the audit and the preparation of the auditor's report.

Standards of Fieldwork

4. The auditor must adequately plan the work and must properly supervise any assistants.

5. The auditor must obtain a sufficient understanding of the entity and its environment, including its internal control, to assess the risk of material misstatement of the financial statements whether due to error or fraud, and to design the nature, timing, and extent of further audit procedures.

6. The auditor must obtain sufficient appropriate audit evidence by performing audit procedures to afford a reasonable basis for an opinion regarding the financial statements under audit.

Standards of Reporting

7. The auditor must state in the auditor's report whether the financial statements are presented in accordance with generally accepted accounting principles.

8. The auditor must identify in the auditor's report those circumstances in which such principles have not been consistently observed in the current period in relation to the preceding period.

9. If the auditor determines that informative disclosures in the financial statements are not reasonably adequate, the auditor must so state in the auditor's report.

10. The auditor's report must either express an opinion regarding the financial statements, taken as a whole, or state that an opinion cannot be expressed. When the auditor cannot express an overall opinion, the auditor should state the reasons in the auditor's report. In all cases where an auditor's name is associated with financial statements, the auditor should clearly indicate the character of the auditor's work, if any, and the degree of responsibility the auditor is taking, in the auditor's report.

Exhibit 6.2

Standard Auditor's Report:
Example of an Unqualified Audit Opinion[4]

"We have audited the accompanying balance sheet of XYZ Company as of December 31, 2XXX, and the related statements of income, retained earnings, and cash flows for the year then ended. these financial statements are the responsibility of the company's management. Our responsibility is to express an opinion on these financial statements based on our audit.

"We conducted our audit based on generally accepted auditing standards. those standards require that we plan and perform the audit to obtain reasonable assurance about whether the financial statements are free of material misstatement. An audit includes examining, on a test basis, evidence supporting the amounts and disclosures in the financial statements. an audit also includes assessing the accounting principles used and significant estimates made by management as well as evaluating the overall financial statement presentation. We believe that our audit provides a reasonable basis for our opinion.

"In our opinion, the financial statements above present fairly, in all material respects, the financial position of XYZ Company as of December 31, 2XXX, and the results of its operations and its cash flow for the year ended in conformity with generally accepted accounting principles."

---

of the audit and/or the financial statements. When the auditor's reservations are more serious, one of the two following types of opinions are rendered.

2. A *disclaimer of opinion* in which auditors state that they cannot give an opinion because of scope limitations (e.g., the auditor has been precluded from completing certain significant audit procedures) or some other reason (e.g., the auditor is not independent).

3. An *adverse opinion* in which the auditors state that the financial statements do not fairly present the financial position of the company, the results of its operations, and the cash flows. In this case, it is claimed that the client is making a serious departure from GAAP.

Types of Auditors

There are three types of auditors generally involved in the various audit examinations: independent (external), internal, and government auditors.

Independent (External) Auditors

The audits of financial statements are performed by independent accountants, usually CPAs. Also, the fact that CPAs are independent, that is, they do not hold an ownership interest or have management involvement in the clients they audit, lends the utmost credibility to their attestations.

Internal Auditors

Unlike independent auditors, internal auditors are employed within the organization and only perform services for that firm. Internal auditors conduct operational and compliance audits for their employer. Essentially, their role is to determine whether the organization and its employees are complying with established policies and procedures and the efficiency and effectiveness of some aspect of the organization's operational activities.

As employees, they lack the degree of independence external auditors possess. However, they usually report to the governing body or to some committee of the board of directors. As medical groups grow in size and scope of operations, it is likely that more groups, especially those that are part of large integrated systems, will employ internal auditors to conduct compliance types of audits and reviews. It is prudent to present all internal audit work product to legal counsel to establish attorney client privilege.

Government Auditors

Government auditors conduct audits under the auspices of various governmental agencies such as the General Accounting Office and the IRS. They usually perform compliance audits to evaluate whether federal laws and regulations are being followed.

Reviews and Compilations of Unaudited Financial Statements

There are two other types of services besides financial statement audits that independent external auditors perform: (1) a review or (2) a compilation of unaudited financial statements. In either case, the work performed is not an audit and should not be construed as equivalent to an independent audit.

Review

In a review, the auditor is trying to provide limited assurance about the fairness of the company's financial statements. Two procedures performed by the accountant in a review engagement beyond those normally required in a compilation are *inquiries of client personnel* and *analytical procedures*. Inquiries relate to the client's use of accounting principles, practices and procedures, and actions taken by meetings of stockholders, key stakeholders and the board of directors that may affect the financial statements. Analytical procedures will normally consist of comparing components of the financial statements with components of comparable prior periods and with budgets and forecasts. The report on reviewed financial statements does express a limited (or negative) assurance statement that "we are not aware of any material modifications that should be made…for them to be in conformity with GAAP."[5]

Compilation

A compilation is the lowest level of service that an independent CPA may perform with respect to financial statements. In a compilation, the accountant merely assembles (or assists the entity in assembling) financial statements. No assurance is provided in a compilation engagement; thus, the accountant cannot issue an opinion or provide any other form of assurance regarding the compiled financial statements.

Obviously, many accountants who issue compilation reports have done much more with their clients' financial statements than simply read them. Accounting standards require that accountants make inquiries or perform additional procedures if they become aware of or suspect that the financial statements could be incomplete, incorrect, or misleading. In addition, for medical practices that are usually smaller, accounting firms often maintain the general ledger and issue compilation reports on the related computerized interim and annual financial statements.

Considerations in Selecting Level of Service

Although an audit provides the most assurance, it is usually much more expensive than a review or compilation. Many practices that have an audit do so because their creditors, investors, or a regulatory body require it.

The middle level of service, the review, generally costs less than an audit but more than a compilation. Although a review does not provide the level of assurance that an audit does, the fact that the outside accountant performs inquiries and analytical procedures is an important consideration. A study of some of the more notorious accounting scandals concluded that these frauds would have been discovered sooner had the auditors done a better job of using simple analytical procedures.[6] The review may be an appropriate level of service for a practice that prepares its financial statements internally but is not required to have an audit. It provides a check on the practice's financial reports, but at a lower cost.

A compilation is usually the least expensive level of service. Although a compilation provides no assurance on the financial statements, it does offer a mechanism for ensuring that the practice's financial data is arranged in proper financial statement format and is accompanied by an outside accountant's report.

Tax Services

Accountants provide a variety of tax services, most of which can be classified as either compliance or planning. Tax compliance includes the preparation of various tax returns and information returns and advising clients of due dates and tax payments in accordance with the various tax laws of federal, state, and local governments. Accountants often represent their clients, usually for an additional fee, in the event a return is audited.

When performing tax planning, the accountant assists clients in arranging their transactions, business structure, and affairs in such a manner as to legally minimize their tax liability. Examples of tax planning include advice selecting the appropriate form of entity; structuring the timing, depreciation, and financing arrangements for asset acquisitions; and year-end tax planning.

Often, an outside accountant will prepare both the entity returns and the owners' individual returns. This helps facilitate tax planning, as physician-owned practices often have multiple related-party transactions. As advisor for both the business and the individual, the accountant gains a better understanding of the clients' total financial state of affairs. Conversely, some groups follow a policy of not using the same accountant for group matters that any group member uses personally. This can help avoid real or perceived conflicts; larger groups will inevitably have physicians who do not use the same accountant as the group.

Other Services

Because of their knowledge of practice operations gained from performing the basic tax and accounting services, accountants are often well-positioned to provide other services to their clients. For example, accountants frequently provide ongoing consulting on an as-needed basis, such as for advice regarding projections, contract negotiations, budgets, profitability studies, capital purchases, strategic planning and other financial matters. Outside accountants who develop a relationship with a particular practice are not just familiar with that particular practice, they have the benefit of knowledge gained from their experiences with other medical groups and businesses in general.

Some accountants have developed niches in certain industries and areas. For example, many provide retirement plan administration, personal financial planning, or business valuation services. Some firms have developed an expertise in healthcare consulting and may perform billing audits, facilitate strategic planning, and carry out other such services.

Some CPAs obtain specialist designations from the AICPA by completing certain education and experience requirements and passing a comprehensive exam. Only CPAs are eligible for these credentialing programs. These include the Personal Financial Specialist, Certified Information Technology Professional, and Accredited in Business Valuation.

A forensic accountant specializes in investigating fraud. The Association of Certified Fraud Examiners confers the Certified Fraud Examiner credential on individuals who meet certain academic and experience requirements and pass a comprehensive exam.

Fraud and Theft

The development and monitoring of internal financial control processes is a critical component of the operational audit portfolio. The operations that support the movement of revenue and accounts payable (A/P) through the practice provides the potential for fraud and theft by employees at multiple points in the process. A number of effective management techniques can minimize the potentially severe impacts of internal fraud and abuse.

Why do employees steal? While experts say that reasons for economic crime in the workplace are numerous, most agree that human greed is at the heart of the problem. Also, the combination of temptation and opportunity offers a formula that can translate to significant losses. The problem probably goes much deeper. These other factors seem to play a role too:

- Lax hiring policies;
- Insufficient checks and balances
- Lack of dual control for cash handling procedures

- Lack of proper management of sample or stocked medications that may have a street value or diverted for personal use of employees or their families.
- Allowing long-time employees easy access to money and products;
- A corporate attitude that appears resigned to a certain amount of crime; and
- Executives who project a callous and uncaring attitude toward employees.

Virtually all individuals who steal from an employer believe that the company is big and profitable and can afford the loss. If you factor in the ease with which employees can manipulate and remove information from some accounting or financial records, then the potential for loss is enormous.

Some Precursors of Fraud and Theft

Certain conditions within medical groups could lead to employee fraud and theft. Recognizing and altering these conditions can deter abusive practices and strengthen the overall framework of control and ethical behavior.

Accounting Systems and Procedures

Many potential trouble spots arise with handling cash, inventory control, supply rooms, and tampering with the accounting system. Here are some samples of poor procedures:

- The same person handles cash receipts and has access to accounts receivable records. In some cases, this individual also deposits the checks at the bank.
- The individual who writes checks for payments also reconciles the bank statements.
- The purchase of goods and services is incompletely documented with purchase authorizations, receiving slips, and vendor invoices, and transactions are not

independently verified by examining these documents before payment is made.

- Physical safeguards are poor and there are no limitations on persons who can access drugs and medical supplies.
- An annual audit of the financial statements and underlying accounting records by an independent auditor is not required or at least one annual independent review does not occur.
- Credit card information that patients have provided for regular payments on their accounts is easily accessed.
- No auditing process for the downloading of patient demographic information

Operations

Several areas involving the staffing and implementation of group activities may indicate ethical weaknesses, such as the following:

- There is heavy employee turnover, particularly at the financial manager position. For example, if there have been three or four different financial managers over a two or three-year period, it could be a sign that senior management is manipulating the books.
- There are large payments made for miscellaneous purposes or services, or unusual patterns in employee expense claims, such as travel or expenditures of a personal nature.
- Employees do not take vacations or time off, especially the financial manager or staff working in finance, and other staff members are not cross trained in the finance areas.
- Employees remain in cash handling or financial management positions when opportunities of advancement have been made.

Management Caricatures

Certain characteristics of physician managers and nonphysician managers might provide an indication of possible misconduct, such as the following:

- Unrealistic performance goals, such as large increases in net income, are set, which drive financial managers to fraudulent practices. These might include creating fictional financial reports, collusion with outside payers, and falsifying records to support erroneous transactions.
- Managers assume clerical functions, such as insisting on personally reconciling all bank statements.
- Managers are unable to find missing records that document large transactions or a series of relatively small transactions.
- Physician-owners display a lackadaisical attitude or uncaring concern for anything financial or financially related to the practice.

Measures to Prevent Fraud and Theft

Faced with the increase in unethical conduct, healthcare entities are taking many preventive measures to deter fraudulent activities. The following sections outline some of these measures.

Tightening the Hiring Process

The effort to decrease employee theft begins with the hiring process. Medical groups can weed out potential thieves in these ways:

- Conduct a complete and probing personal interview of each applicant.
- Contact previous places of employment to verify dates of employment and positions held.
- Consider credit history on cash handling and financial management staff
- Check with the candidate's university or professional school to see if the person actually graduated.
- Interview personal references very thoroughly by asking tough follow-up questions.
- Conduct complete background checks on providers and higher-level managers to be hired.

- Develop your own references for candidates for high-level positions.

Strengthening Deterrents

Every business, including medical groups, should have an ethics policy and a published and prominent standard of conduct for all group members to follow. The policy and code should stipulate what constitutes illegal and irregular activities as well as the consequences of such actions. Furthermore, the physician-owners and top management should set the example by displaying proper behavior that typifies ethical conduct.

With this proper overall framework, other deterrent actions might consist of the following:

- Establish a strong system of accountability among the members of the governing body in which they must answer fully for their actions and the fulfillment of their responsibilities.
- Devise methods to keep all members of the governing body informed in a clear, concise, and current manner about the activities of the medical group. Make sure those with less training or experience understand the financial impacts of all decisions regarding the organization.
- Designate certain members of the governing body who have some financial experience to be the prime monitors of the financial statements and reports prepared by the financial manager and/or the staff.
- Set up a budgetary control system that physicians and other managers can understand. The system should embrace the operating budget and long-term capital budget. Both budgets should be subject to the scrutiny of top management and the governing body of the medical group. Create a culture of accountability if budgets are under or over preforming.
- Insist that professional service contracts be explicit as to what is to be provided, how it is to be paid for, and what

supporting documentation will be part of the contract. Do not permit the submission of documents that read "for X hours of service" as the only support for payment.

- Develop clear and precise compensation model that are easy to explain and produce. Each provider should be able to explain their compensation model in detail.

- Create a compensation philosophy that recommends compensation models, adjustments to the model and are benchmarked.

- Create a compensation committee who can advise and monitor the compensation model assuring that goals of the model is are being achieve and make adjustments if they are not.

- Encourage a positive attitude toward the medical group by treating all employees fairly and openly and making sure that human relations policies are supportive of employee rights and concerns.

- Provide adequate compensation levels and employee benefits comparable to other healthcare entities in the local area so employees are less likely to feel taken advantage of and possibly wanting to seek retribution.

Establishing Conflict-of-Interest Restrictions

Many practices today require all employees to sign conflict-of-interest statements promising they will not take advantage of an outside interest to profit illegally from the company. While this may not yet be a practice followed by medical groups, the time has arrived to consider such a policy for the physicians and managers of the group. For example, if someone in the group has an interest in an outside business not necessarily connected with direct medical care services but which provides a service to the group, that relationship is immediately suspect, especially if it is not openly revealed. Also, when a member of the group — physician, nonphysician provider, or manager — is doing business with a longtime friend or relative, the group member should remain objective and insist on having detailed contracts and underlying documentation. These data should be scrutinized by other members of the group to ensure that transactions are appropriate and sanctioned by group management.

Installing and Continuously Updating Computer Security Systems

A growing proportion of business fraud is committed via the computer. Management must be alert and should use the latest electronic security tools. The most important preventive controls are those that limit access to computers, data files, programs, and system documentation to a minimum number of persons. Methods of limiting access include defining employee duties, segregating functional responsibilities, dual-person access, enforced vacations for personnel, physical security, and electronic surveillance and security, including access-code passwords. Governing bodies of medical groups should use outside consultants who specialize in security password control, networking security, and other key elements of computer security to establish and make sure the latest measures are in effect.

Protecting the Medical Group Itself

Sometimes as part of the standard business insurance package, *employee dishonesty insurance* protects the business against losses from employee theft. To add this coverage, the insurers may need to check the group's hiring procedures and theft-prevention efforts.

In addition, employers can buy fidelity bonds to cover all employees or only certain positions, such as bookkeepers or financial managers or specifically named employees.

Confronting and Prosecuting Offenders

When carrying out policies and procedures aimed at stopping fraud and theft, medical group management must confront violators openly and in a straightforward manner. Ignoring these violations or excusing such actions sends the wrong message to other employees and destroys the tone that top management should be setting for all to act honestly and legally. There must be strong and visible evidence of a commitment to ethics and moral behavior in all aspects of the group's activities. Some helpful hints to reinforce these ideas include:

- Do not tolerate harassment at any level of the organization, particularly at the top. There should be no bending of the rules or ignoring them since such action will likely lead to a degeneration of the rules of proper conduct. You should review harassment tolerance in annual employee training classes.
- Pay attention to stress factors that key staff members may display. To avert possible misappropriation by stressed individuals, intervene when it is in the best interest of the group by offering assistance to the person in whatever manner is deemed necessary.
  - Consider contracting with an employee assistance service vendor to assist employees dealing with personal and professional stress. You should consider allowing family members of employees the same opportunity to access the service.
- Do not compromise on carrying out professional and personal ethics. If a problem exists with an individual, assist in finding a solution even if there is some discomfort experienced by the participants.
  - Management should be trained to detect when an employee is acting out of character and in intervention techniques that they can implement to assist employees.
- Create a culture where employees feel welcome to discuss their problems without being judged or exposed to employment sanctions.

While it seems humane to refrain from prosecuting violators of ethical conduct, aggressive prosecution can also send a strong warning to anyone else who is stealing or conspiring with others. Medical group managers must be determined to reduce theft with a broad program of surveillance, security, and, where necessary, prosecution of offenders.

In the final analysis, financial decision making depends on the integrity of the financial manager. Groups must have in place management and staff with ethical and moral values and the strength necessary to act within a defined set of rules that are appropriate in our society. Leadership is needed to display personal character and courage because without it, we will not have ethical behavior in any of our institutions.

Internal Control of Cash

An internal control process safeguards the assets of the practice; provides for reliable and accurate information; and ensures compliance with organizational objectives, policies, and procedures. Medical groups have reported that one of the most important objectives of a financial information system is to provide proper internal control over cash. This is intended to:

- Establish custody over cash;
- Protect cash from fraud or theft;
- Limit the temptation of otherwise honest employees; and
- Provide a check on accuracy and reliability of cash records.

The internal control of cash requires a fairly extensive and concentrated series of procedures. The following discussion highlights some of the more popular methods of establishing internal control over cash.

Employee Screening and Training

The practice may wish to use background testing as a means to assess ethical behavior and competency of candidates. Criminal background checks are useful in screening out candidates with known criminal backgrounds, but they will not eliminate all dishonest employees. You also may want to consider credit history checks on applicants.

Ethics Training

Medical practices might reduce the potential for fraud by providing ethics training to their employees. The *2012 Report to the Nations on Occupational Fraud and Abuse* by the Association of Certified Fraud Examiners (ACFE) found that while all internal controls contributed to reduced losses, formal management reviews, employee support programs, and hotlines for reporting suspicions were correlated with the greatest decreases in financial losses.

Segregation of Duties

An effective internal control process requires that cash functions be divided among personnel in such a manner that makes embezzlement or mishandling or theft of cash more difficult. This means that employees with cash functions should not perform incompatible functions, so responsibilities for handling cash, recording transactions, and authorizing transactions should be separated. No one person should have complete authority over the entire sequence of transactions that involve cash (e.g., from the purchase of a resource through payment).

Smaller offices sometimes have difficulty achieving good separation of duties. A practice can often achieve appropriate segregation of duties by expanding some responsibilities beyond the core administrative staff. For example, the practice might use physicians, or nonphysician providers, non-administrative staff, or outside accountants to perform certain functions. Having physicians or nonphysician providers perform a large number of administrative tasks may not be productive if it reduces the time available to see patients and produce revenue. However, having physician-owners perform some tasks, such as dropping off the bank deposit, might allow them to more effectively provide oversight of practice management and operations.

The general theory regarding segregation of duties is shown in Exhibit 6.3. For cash, the two primary areas requiring segregation of duties are (1) cash receipts and (2) cash disbursements.

254

Exhibit 6.3
Segregation of Duties (General Theory)[7]

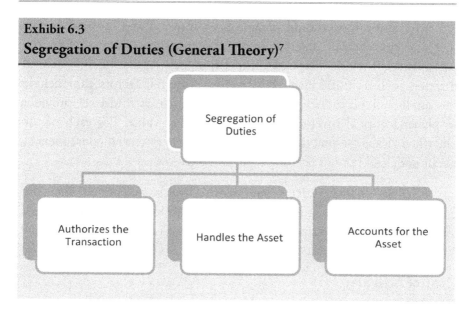

Risk Assessment

Before a practice can determine which controls to implement as part of its internal control process, it must first identify the risks that would prevent the practice from reaching its goals in operations, financial reporting, and compliance. For example:

- Employees stealing from incoming cash could prevent a practice from reaching its targeted profitability;

- An incompetent financial manager might not produce reliable financial statements, thus misrepresenting the practice's financial position and results of operations;

- A coder might overcode evaluation and management codes, resulting in an Office of Inspector General, U.S. Department of Health and Human Services audit and financial penalties; and

- Information systems that lack proper security are accessible to outside hackers.

Risk assessment should include both internal and external factors that can prevent the practice from achieving its objectives.[8] External factors might include increased competition, new legislation, or a natural disaster, such as hurricanes or tornadoes. Internal factors can include the quality of personnel, a disruptive physician or mid-level provider, or pharmaceutical inventory with a high street value. For each of the identified risks, the practice should estimate the potential consequences, likelihood, and how to best manage the risk.

Finally, change affects an organization's objectives and the environment in which it operates. Thus, a practice needs to be forward looking in its risk assessment, provide a mechanism for identifying new risks, and reassess its risks on a regular basis.[9]

Control Activities

After the practice identifies its risks, it must determine how it will mitigate those risks. Because each practice has its own unique personnel, location, and operational issues, no one set of controls will work for every practice. However, certain controls, such as safeguarding cash and segregating duties, are available to all businesses.

Control activities must fit the practice's operations. For example, a large family practice group will typically need tight controls over the cash collected from patients at the time of visit, such as copayments and deductibles. Conversely, pathology practices do not generally see or collect any money from patients; consequently, they would not require cash drawers and would not need policies for time-of-service collections.

Policies and Procedures

Controls often take the form of policies and procedures, training and annual review, which formalize the rules, identify the consequences for breaking the rules, and provide uniform discipline and consequences. Because policies and procedures support management actions and spell them out, employees are warned that they cannot avoid punishment if caught, which reduces the probability of inappropriate activity.

Particularly in cases of *gray area* frauds, such as acceptance of small gifts from vendors or personal use of office supplies, policies and procedures can educate employees about the difference between right and wrong. Acknowledgment and understanding of the policy and procedures provides indirect ethics training to staff members and helps create a more effective control environment.

Physical Controls

Physical controls provide barriers to accessing assets. For example, a practice might lock its medical supplies and drugs in a closet and provide a key only to designated individuals. Most organizations keep cash locked in a safe or cash drawer. And making sure only certain authorized individuals have access to the practice after hours is a physical control.

Information System Controls

Like most businesses today, almost all medical practices use computers to process information. Thus, information system controls are an important part of a practice's internal control process. For medical practices, information system controls are necessary not only to help meet financial and operational goals, but they are also necessary to ensure compliance with HIPAA security rules. Computer and program passwords and differing security settings are very common information system controls.

Preventive and Detective Controls

In evaluating internal controls, the administrator should consider both preventive and detective controls. *Preventive controls* prevent an undesirable event from happening. For example, requiring computer passwords which each employee is required to change at certain time intervals is a preventive control because passwords prevent access to programs and data by users who don't know the password, and they create an audit trail for authorized users. Additionally, having daily data backups on-site as well as off-site is a sound preventive control measure.

Detective controls detect an undesirable event after it has happened. For example, reconciling a bank account is a detective control because the person balancing the bank account could detect unusual transactions when reconciling the account. The reconciliation does not prevent the undesirable events from happening, but it should detect them after they happen. Preventive controls are generally more effective and less expensive than detective controls, but both have a place in the internal control process.

Cost-Effectiveness

Another factor to consider when establishing controls is the cost-effectiveness of the control. For example, an ophthalmology practice with an extensive inventory of eyewear for resale might determine that a computerized inventory control system would be cost effective. Conversely, for a practice with a minimal amount of supplies, that program would be likely to cost more than any savings from improved oversight. Although control activities in small offices are less formal than in a larger office, they are still effective because management oversight and communication with employees may be more direct.

Internal Control over Cash Receipts

Specific individuals in the group should be designated to handle and be responsible for cash. Others should not be permitted to do so. Furthermore, the practice should segregate the functions relating to cash receipts to ensure that the individuals who handle cash and checks do not post the payments and related adjustments, and still another individual performs the bank reconciliation.

Accounting records must be kept by persons who do not handle or have access to cash. Front office staff should not be permitted to record transactions in patient accounts receivable, and accountants responsible for receivables should not physically handle cash receipts or payment.

Finally, still another person should be responsible for reconciling the bank account. This person should not handle cash or post the accounting records.

The suggested segregation of duties over cash receipts is shown in Exhibit 6.4.

Other tips regarding control over cash receipts include:

- Medical billing software generally allows for assigning staff members access to various functions. Make sure that those employees who receive cash receipts are not allowed access to the payment posting and adjustment functions.
- Maximize use of bank lockboxes and electronic payments to minimize the amount of cash that is physically in the office. This enhances segregation of duties by avoiding office staff access to that cash.
- If your practice receives checks from patients and insurance companies in the mail, consider having two staff members open the mail together.
- One way to expedite the deposit of checks into the practice's bank account is to use a check-scanning machine at the office that transmits the check information to the bank for electronic deposit. To further eliminate the potential for embezzlement or misplacement of the

Exhibit 6.4
Segregation of Duties for Cash Receipts[10]

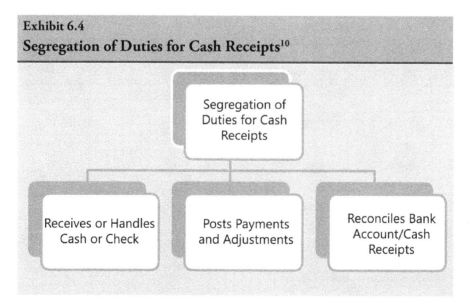

check, have the checkout personnel scan the check in front of patients and give them their receipts at that time.

- All cash receipts should be deposited intact daily. No payments should be made out of undeposited cash receipts. Only the petty cash or change fund should remain on the premises overnight.
- A verifiable record should be made immediately after each cash receipt, such as a remittance advice.

Internal Control over Cash Disbursements

The practice should ensure proper segregation of duties among employees with cash disbursement functions. Exhibit 6.5 shows the suggested segregation of duties for cash disbursements personnel.

The functions of authorizing disbursements, preparing checks and maintaining the A/P records, signing checks, and mailing or distributing checks should be performed by different individuals. Yet another person with no other cash disbursement responsibilities should reconcile the bank account. In some smaller practices, the functions of signing checks and authorizing transactions are combined. While it is important for the check signer to review the supporting documentation for all of the checks

Exhibit 6.5

Segregation of Duties for Cash Disbursements[11]

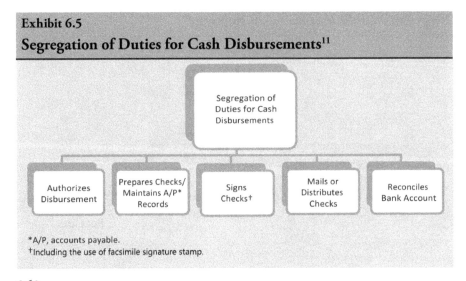

*A/P, accounts payable.
†Including the use of facsimile signature stamp.

that he or she signs, it is especially important for check signers who bear the sole responsibility for authorizing transactions.

In some practices, especially smaller groups, the physicians may give check-signing responsibility to a trusted employee who also prepares the checks, mails or distributes them, and maintains the A/P records.

Sometimes this person even reconciles the bank account. Such practices violate the recommended segregation of duties and leave the practice vulnerable to embezzlement, even when such employees have never committed such offenses in the past. A 2012 ACFE study revealed that only 8 percent of employees who committed occupational fraud had been previously convicted of a fraud-related offense.[12] The important thing to remember is that every criminal commits a first crime. The failure of a practice to institute recommended internal controls could provide the temptation that leads an honest employee to becoming a dishonest employee.

Many people unfamiliar with best practices for accounting ask why it is necessary for the mailing or delivery of checks to be performed by a separate person. It may seem like common sense to give these documents back to the A/P clerk to mail since the A/P clerk maintains those records and should seemingly be able to perform this function most effectively. The problem with this scenario is that a signed check is a cash equivalent. A dishonest A/P clerk who performs both of these functions might prepare checks payable to bogus vendors or open up personal checking accounts in the name of legitimate vendors and misappropriate checks payable to those vendors. He or she might prepare checks with the intention of changing the payee or amount. These frauds would be much more difficult to perpetrate if the A/P clerk does not receive the signed checks to mail and distribute.

For these reasons and more, the recommended workflow for cash disbursements is:

1. An approved employee should hold the responsibility to verify and authorize invoice payment;

2. The A/P clerk processes the checks and gives them to a physician or administrator for signature;

3. The physician or administrator signs them and gives them to another employee to mail; and

4. Another executive, administrator, or financial employee reconciles the bank account.

Beware of Facsimile Signature Stamps

Some practices use facsimile signature stamps of legitimate check signers' signatures to sign checks. While this practice may be convenient when the authorized check signer is a busy physician or works in another location, it is a risky practice that can weaken internal control over the cash disbursements function. A person who has access to the facsimile signature stamps should have no other function in the cash disbursement process. The stamp should be stored in a secure location such as a safe and locked drawer. Additionally, as part of the auditing process you should know how many stamps exist for each signer. For example, this person should not be responsible for preparing or mailing A/P checks. Even though this individual is technically not an authorized check signer, this person does have the ability to provide an authorized signature on a check. Practices should seriously consider eliminating facsimile signature stamps.

Electronic Payments

Most practices make their payments electronically. For example, many tax payments are required to be made in this manner. In addition, some vendors may require that payments be made electronically. In other cases, the terms for timing of payment may be so narrow that payments made sending a paper check through the mail could lead to potential late charges and/or finance charges. The practice should ensure segregation of duties with regard to the electronic payments just as it should for paper checks. Many banks allow for dual controls on automated clearinghouse (ACH) payments, which let one individual initiate a transaction and another approve the transaction.

Other Controls over Cash Disbursements

Medical groups should also use the following internal controls related to cash disbursements:

- Cash disbursements should be made by check or by bank ACH, unless specifically authorized from petty cash.
- The checks should be prenumbered, and the stock of blank checks should be kept under adequate safeguards with access given only to persons authorized to sign checks.
- Voided checks should be destroyed. If the group prefers to save these, then it should (1) tear out the signature portion of the check and (2) keep them under safeguards similar to blank checks.
- No payments should be made without proper authorization and verification of the amounts due. When checks are signed, the signer should have all supporting documentation available for review to ensure that the disbursements are valid and appropriate. Some practices may consider dual signatures on their checks, but with proper controls this may be unnecessary.

Restrict Credit Card Access

Restrict the use of company debit or credit cards. Giving someone a credit or debit card is similar to giving that person access to cash. Consider an expense reimbursement or expense advance situation as an alternative. Remember that when an employee requests a check, practice management has the ability to review the documentation and refuse the request. With the cards, the practice is liable for these disbursements without the right to review the documentation in advance to determine the legitimacy of the business purpose for the disbursement. Furthermore, getting the related copies of invoices, receipts and other documentation after the charge is made can sometimes be difficult. Credit and debit cards further increase the risk that personal, unauthorized, or otherwise inappropriate expenses will be incurred by the practice.

Some financial institutions issue credit cards that can be set up to allow only certain classifications of expenditures to be made using the cards. Management generally has the ability to determine which types of expenditures will be allowed. Practices that use credit cards should consider using cards that offer these types of controls. Depending on the level of management, consider limiting the amount available on the credit and debit card. You should also consider limiting travel and purchases expense by management level staff.

General Cash Controls

Some recommended general controls are as follows:

- For the protection of the medical group, the cashier and others who handle cash regularly should be bonded. However, the practice may be able to reduce premiums and obtain the equivalent protection by adding an employee dishonesty or employee theft endorsement to the policy.
- Cash balances should be verified daily through the daily cash report and review of bank activity over the internet.
- By reviewing work areas and trash, it may become apparent that duplicate records, logs, or separate receipt books are being kept.
- Having a substitute perform office functions for a vacationing employee may uncover improprieties in the receivables or charges. Rotating duties without notice and separating functions will reduce the opportunities for embezzlement.
- Make sure to investigate any patient complaints about billing errors or omissions. A fraudulent person may hold open a deposit waiting for a replacement payment or skim from a deposit if the office does not reconcile the deposits to the bank statements. The administrator should follow up on any unusual or suspicious comparisons and randomly review charge entry or scheduled encounter forms against the billed charges, adjustments, and received payments for any discrepancies.

- Limiting access by passwords or administrative function will reduce the opportunities for inappropriate recording of charges, payments or write-offs.
- When a resignation of cash handling or financial management employee is received, consider performing an audit prior to their departure and immediately after. All user access, passwords or internet rights to IT, A/R, and A/P functions should be removed immediately upon departure.

Information and Communication

Communication is crucial to a system of internal controls. The practice should ensure that it identifies, captures, and communicates *relevant* information in a timely and effective format. Doing so is essential for management, employees, the board of directors, and other stakeholders to properly carry out their responsibilities.

Employees need to know how to manage their responsibilities in the practice's internal control process. They must understand the organization's risks and how their responsibilities fit into the entire internal control process because frontline employees are often in a good position to recognize new risks and problems.

Communication plays an important role in detecting fraud. ACFE data from 2012 indicates that 43.3 percent of frauds were detected by a tip, which is more than by any other method and nearly three times the percentage detected by an external audit. A majority (50.9 percent) of those tips came from employees, 22.1 percent came from customers, 12.4 percent were anonymous, and 9.0 percent came from vendors. Some of the tips were received via a hotline, while others were the result of management maintaining open channels of communications with employees, vendors, and customers.[13]

Larger practices might consider hotlines, third party managed hotline, or web-based portals as mechanisms for reducing the incidence of fraud. ACFE 2012 data indicate that hotlines have an interesting effect on how fraud is discovered. In organizations without hotlines, more

265

than 11 percent of fraud was caught by accident; if the organization had a hotline, only 3 percent of fraud was accidentally discovered.[14]

Communication between management and employees is usually easier and more frequent in a smaller organization with fewer levels of organizational hierarchy and more opportunities for management to interact with the employees. No matter the techniques a medical practice uses to report fraud, the employee reporting must believe it is confidential if they choose to remain anonymous. It also must not impact their employment status. It is also essential that, until proven through extensive audit, every employee deserves the opportunity to explain the circumstances of a reported fraud. Additionally, in order to maintain an effective hotline, employees must be given a level of confidence that their reporting was investigated and changes were implemented. Under no situation shall the person making the report know the outcome of the investigation on another employee.

Monitoring Internal Controls

Once a practice has implemented its system of internal control, it needs to monitor the system to ensure that it continues to operate effectively. This can be achieved by ongoing monitoring activities or a separate evaluation.

Ongoing Monitoring Activities

The practice can obtain ongoing assessment of its internal control process by building ongoing monitoring activities into its normal operating activities. For example:

- In carrying out their managerial functions and the audit process, managers can spot inconsistent information, unusual trends, cash counts that are out of balance, and checks that have been altered;
- When following up on complaints from vendors and patients, problems can be uncovered; and
- Training and planning meetings can provide feedback on the effectiveness of the internal control process.

Many management activities, such as review of financial or operational data and being alert to what occurs in the practice on a day-to-day basis, are ongoing monitoring activities. Other ongoing monitoring activities are regular reports on the system of internal control (completed by internal or external auditors) and periodic statements by personnel regarding the code of conduct, compliance, and other issues affecting internal control.

Insiders or outsiders should perform separate evaluations and approach these activities as a "fresh look" rather than as a regular audit or ongoing review of an existing process. Examples of separate evaluation methodologies are checklists, questionnaires, flowcharts, and matrix analyses.

One tool that has been developed since the Committee of Sponsoring Organizations of the Treadway Commission (COSO) study is the control self-assessment (CSA). This methodology, developed by CPA firms and some of the professional organizations that sponsored the COSO study, is a tool for insiders to use to evaluate their organization's internal control. The Institute of Internal Auditors offers CSA certification and has developed extensive literature and information about this process. One survey of organizations that had performed a CSA found that the companies often achieved process improvements as a by-product of the CSA, confirming the COSO view of internal control as a process.[15]

The scope and frequency of separate evaluations will depend on the practice's risks and other attributes. For example, the COSO study indicated that special evaluations may not be as necessary in smaller and mid-size organizations. In these organizations, management is typically more involved in the day-to-day operations and is therefore more likely to become aware of internal control problems on an informal basis.[16]

Separate Evaluation

A separate evaluation is an unbiased look at the internal control system that is carried on outside of the practice's normal business operations. This evaluation is a planned process as opposed to a series of random, mechanical tests. It can be done by internal or external parties.

Smaller organizations often have better ongoing monitoring than larger organizations, because management often has direct knowledge of problems and potential issues with customers, vendors, and regulators. Smaller practices are less likely to engage in separate evaluations and may already have highly effective ongoing monitoring activities.

The Fraud Triangle

These three factors must all be present for a trust violation to occur:

1. A financial need that is non-shareable (i.e., motivation);

2. Perceived opportunity; and

3. Rationalization.

Common types of fraud include:

Skimming. In a skimming scheme, the perpetrator simply takes the money before it is recorded on the organization's books. The perpetrator may either skim revenue, supplies, or assets.

Lapping. This is a receivables skimming scheme where an embezzler misappropriates a payment from Patient A, posts a payment from Patient B to Patient A's account, posts a payment from Patient C to Patient B's account, and so forth, until the perpetrator pays back all the patients' accounts, the scheme is uncovered, or another form of fraud is used to cover the embezzler's tracks.

Cash larceny. This is stealing incoming cash after it has been recorded on the books, which often involves destroying or falsifying records.

Bogus refunds. The embezzler creates an overpayment on a patient's account and uses it to issue him or herself a refund check.

Simple cash disbursements fraud. This involves check tampering and other misuse of checks. Fraud perpetrators use a variety of methods to divert practice funds for personal purposes. Whether they commit the crime by obtaining a legitimate or forged signature, forging an endorsement, or altering the check, they must usually falsify accounting records to conceal their fraud.

Obtaining a signature. For some perpetrators, obtaining a signature is not a problem because they either are authorized check signers or have access to a facsimile signature stamp. Yet another group of such criminals forge the signature of an authorized check signer on the check. The perpetrator might also alter the check after it is signed, as discussed next.

Forged endorsements. Some dishonest employees forge the endorsement on checks made out to legitimate vendors and pocket the cash.

Altering checks. Checks are altered after they have been signed.

Counterfeiting checks. Some dishonest employees may copy the legitimate checks of the practice or another individual, often by using a scanner. By scanning a signed check, the perpetrator also obtains copies of authorized signatures.

Pay-and-return scams. The perpetrator intentionally overpays a vendor and pockets the returned payment.

Bogus expense reimbursements. Perpetrators of this type of fraud seek bogus reimbursement for personal expenses or inflate the amounts of legitimate business expenses. The expense reports may be accompanied by altered or insufficient support documents. In the expense-report version of the pay-and-return scheme, the fraudsters may claim reimbursement on returned merchandise or air tickets or submit multiple requests for reimbursement for the same expense.

Credit card fraud. This involves charging personal expenses on cards or failing to turn in the appropriate documentation for legitimate card purchases.

Shell company schemes. An employee pays a fictitious business for goods or services never received. The fictitious businesses are usually listed as owned by the employee, relatives, or accomplices.

Pass-through schemes. The practice actually receives goods or services from the vendor at an inflated price. This type of scheme involves a fraudulent intermediary who purchases supplies from a legitimate vendor and sells them to the practice at an inflated price.

Kickback schemes. Kickback schemes involve off-the-books payments by vendors to employees in exchange for the employees influencing business transactions. The line between a legitimate business gift and a corrupt business practice can be fuzzy. (To avoid having to make this distinction, some practices have a policy that prohibits or limits the acceptance of gifts.)

Personal purchases. The purchase of goods and services from legitimate vendors for the perpetrator's personal use or use in his or her side business.

Falsified hours or salary. This is the most common type of payroll fraud. The easiest way to pull off this fraud is to turn in a false timecard. For manual timecards, the perpetrators can accomplish this by forging their supervisor's signature. Another way employees falsify their earnings is to change their rate of pay in the payroll system. Generally, employees who perpetrate this fraud must have access to the payroll system.

Ghost schemes. The corrupt employee causes a paycheck to be issued to a real or fictitious individual (the *ghost*) who does not actually work for the practice. To carry out this scheme, the perpetrator must usually have either hiring authority or access to the payroll records. Consequently, managers are often the usual suspects in a ghost employee scheme.

Misappropriation of supplies and equipment. This involves stealing anything from basic office supplies to major items that would qualify as larceny.

Pharmaceutical theft. This is particularly problematic, not just because of the value of the drugs, but also because of the implications for breaking federal and state laws for narcotics and other controlled substances. Also problematic is prescription fraud, in which the perpetrators alter an existing prescription or forge the physician's name on a new prescription.

Retirement plan fraud. Because these plans often hold a significant amount of investments, they can be lucrative targets for fraud. Typically, practices use third-party custodians and administrators to monitor pension funds so unauthorized access is minimized.

Financial statement fraud. This occurs when an employee or some other insider intentionally falsifies an organization's financial statements.

Technology-related fraud. This can include anything from stealing account-access passwords to using patient information for identity theft.

Internal Control Checklist

Medical groups may have audits performed of their financial statements and, in the process, have their system of internal controls evaluated. An internal controls checklist used by the auditor (Exhibit 6.6) provides an opportunity to review the areas

Exhibit 6.6
Internal Control Checklist[18]

Yes	No	Recommended Practices
		Cash Fund
		Petty cash or change fund maintained (imprest system)
		A custodian is responsible for this fund
		Fund reimbursement is made directly to the custodian
		Custodian has no access to accounting reports
		Custodian has no access to cash receipts
		Physically secure place for fund storage
		Surprise audits conducted periodically
		Rule prohibiting employee check cashing
		Cash Receipts
		All cash receipts deposited daily
		Daily list of mail receipts
		Daily reconciliation of cash collections required
		Cashier personnel separated from accounting functions
		Cashier personnel separated from credit functions
		Cash custodian apart from negotiable instruments
		Bank account properly authorized
		Bank instructed not to cash checks from the clinic to the clinic
		Comparisons made between duplicate deposit slips and detail of accounts receivable
		Comparisons made between duplicate deposit slips and cash book
		Cash Disbursements
		Recording, authorizing, and check-signing activities completely separate
		Support required for check signature
		Control exercised if check-signing machine or facsimile signature stamp used
		Limited authorization to sign checks
		No access to cash records or receipts by check signers
		Detailed listing of checks required
		Check listings compared with cash book
		No checks payable to cash allowed
		Checks are prenumbered
		Physical control over unused checks
		Destruction or mutilation of voided checks required
		All disbursements made by check, unless specifically authorized from cash or ACH
		ACH payments require separate initiation and approval
		Control over and prompt accounting for all electronic payments
		Control over and prompt accounting for interbank transfers
		Bank Reconciliation
		Reconciliation between bank and books conducted at least monthly
		Cash balances should be verified daily through the daily cash report and review of bank activity over the Internet (or other appropriate means)
		Person responsible for reconciling bank statements is independent from accounting or cashier duties
		Bank statement sent directly to the person responsible for reconciliation
		General
		All employees who handle cash are bonded

examined during the evaluation. A "no" response to an item indicates a possible weakness and should be examined for possible modification to improve the internal controls procedures.

Bank Reconciliation

A critical part of control over cash is the reconciliation of every bank account. Because it constitutes the verification of two independent accounting systems, it is important that the bank reconciliation be performed by a person who does not have responsibility for cash or maintaining the related accounting records. These reconciliations should generally be performed by an individual at a high level in the organization, although very small groups may have an outside accountant perform this function. Exhibit 6.7 provides a simplified example of a bank reconciliation. Note that this form provides double proof of the correct cash balance.

In the past, good internal control practices included promptly performing reconciliations on a monthly basis upon receiving bank statements in the mail at the beginning of the month. With the advent of internet banking, practices can reconcile bank balances at any time during the month. Moreover, today's increased frequency of electronic transactions, including both cash receipts and disbursements, makes more frequent review of bank activity and bank reconciliations a recommended practice. No matter the frequency of the reconciliations any discrepancies need to be reported immediately and investigated. Depending on the findings, changes in policies and procedures, employee assignments and new controls may be needed to assure that the issue discovered is contained and no future issues will arise. The degree of the issue may require reporting to senior management, physician owner or key stakeholders.

Internet Banking

Today's fast-paced use of electronic transactions demands that practices use internet banking. Practices are now receiving funds from

Exhibit 6.7
Bank Reconciliation[19]

Balance per Books	$ xxx	Balance per Bank Statement	$ xxx
Add: Amounts that have been added by the bank to the account that have not been recorded on the books (e.g., proceeds from a bank loan)	$xxxx	*Add:* Amounts that have been recorded on the books that have not yet been recorded by the bank (e.g., deposits in transit)	$xxxx
Subtract: Amounts that have been deducted by the bank that have not yet been recorded on the books (e.g., bank service charges)	xxx	*Subtract:* Amounts that have been deducted on the books that have not yet been recorded by the bank (e.g., outstanding checks)	xxx
Corrected balance	$xxxx	Corrected balance	$xxxx

many payers electronically, paying many of their taxes electronically, and paying some vendors electronically. As discussed earlier, practices should be viewing their bank account activity online on an ongoing basis and reconciling their bank balance on an interim basis throughout the month. The increased potential for fraud demands that the practice be vigilant in reviewing this data. Unauthorized or questionable transactions should be reported promptly to the bank, as the time frame for reporting these items and being reimbursed for the related losses may be short. Also, banks may consider a lack of certain internal controls within the practice a sufficient reason for not reimbursing those losses. In connection with the setup and ongoing use of its internet banking function, the practice should be vigilant about internet security. Be very careful about which individuals have access to view bank account information and even more vigilant as to which individuals are given authority to initiate and authorize funds transactions. Have independent individuals with information technology expertise review the security system and protocols of all computers and networks involved in internet banking. The protocols should incorporate the frequency and complexity of passwords, the process for investigating and responding to suspected breaches, and employee training.

One advantage of internet banking is that it can provide owners and executives with better opportunities for oversight of cash functions.

For example, when practices received only a paper bank statement in the mail, the person who received this statement had the potential to alter it or remove damaging evidence, such as unauthorized checks, from the envelope. In contrast, altering or removing the data that appear in the practice's online banking activity would be very difficult, and multiple people can view it — not just the person who has the paper bank statement. Furthermore, if any of the owners are physicians who are busy seeing patients during office hours and have little time for reviewing banking activity, internet banking allows them to view activity from home, thus providing additional oversight over cash.

Conclusion

The effective management of auditing processes ensures the ongoing financial integrity of the medical practice. Key knowledge required to manage the audit process effectively includes understanding the various types of audits and the processes that will be audited, working knowledge of GAAS, determining the need for audits, implementing internal controls, instituting effective relationships with auditing entities, and reporting and follow up of the report findings.

Notes

1. Lawrence Wolper, *Physician Practice Management: Essential Operational and Financial Knowledge*, 2nd ed. (Burlington, MA: Jones & Bartlett Learning, 2012), 498.

2. Wolper, *Physician Practice Management*, 296, 298, 300.

3. "Generally Accepted Auditing Standards," American Institute of Certified Public Accountants (AICPA), page 871, modified November 2006, www.aicpa.org/Research/Standards/AuditAttest/DownloadableDocuments/ AU-00150.pdf.

4. "Generally Accepted Auditing Standards," 871–872.

5. D.R. Carchmichael and Lynford Graham, *Special Industries and Special Topics, vol. 2, Accountants' Handbook*, 12th ed. (Hoboken, NJ: Wiley, 2012), 65.

6. Ray Whittington, *Analytical Procedures for Small Business Engagements*, an AICPA Self-Study Course (Lewisville, TX: American Institute of Certified Public Accountants, 2005).

7. *Financial Management for Medical Groups: A Resource for New and Experienced Managers*, 3rd ed. (Englewood, CO: MGMA, 2014), 231, exhibit 8.5.

8. Committee of Sponsoring Organizations of the Treadway Commission (COSO), *Internal Control: Integrated Framework: Executive Summary*" (Durham, NC: AICPA, May 1, 2013). www.coso.org/documents/990025P_Executive_Summary_final_may20_e.pdf.

9. COSO, *Internal Control*, 43–46.

10. *Financial Management for Medical Groups*, 232, exhibit 8.6.

11. *Financial Management for Medical Groups*, 233, exhibit 8.7.

12. Association of Certified Fraud Examiners (ACFE), *Report to the Nations on Occupational Fraud and Abuse: 2012 Global Study* (Austin, TX: ACFE, Jan. 1, 2012). www.acfe.com/uploadedFiles/ACFE_Website/Content/rttn/2012-report-to-nations.pdf.

13. ACFE, *Report to the Nations on Occupational Fraud and Abuse*, 16.

14. ACFE, *Report to the Nations on Occupational Fraud and Abuse*, 16.

15. William E. Thompson, *Internal Controls: Design and Documentation* (Englewood, CO: MicroMash, 2006).

16. Thompson, *Internal Controls*, 76–77.

17. ACFE, *Report to the Nations on Occupational Fraud and Abuse*, 40.

18. *Financial Management for Medical Groups*, 236, exhibit 8.8.

19. *Financial Management for Medical Groups*, 237, exhibit 8.9.

Resource List

The following resources are available online. Please visit the MGMA Store at www.mgma.org/store for updates and new products. Members of MGMA seeking assistance locating articles and industry resources on financial management may contact the MGMA Knowledge Center at infocenter@mgma.org.

MGMA Books and Reports

Financial Management for Medical Groups: A Resource for New and Experienced Managers, by MGMA (2014).

Get the Money in the Door: Physician Billing Basics, by Sarah J. Holt (2010).

Medical Office Billing: A Self-Study Training Manual, by Sarah J. Holt (2012).

MGMA Chart of Accounts, sixth edition, by MGMA (2014).

The Physician Billing Process: 12 Potholes to Avoid on the Road to Getting Paid, third edition, by Deborah Walker Keegan and Elizabeth W. Woodcock.

RVUs: Applications for medical practice success, third edition, by Frank Cohen (2013).

MGMA Practice Resources Topics and Tools Sections

See the following topic-focused sections on the MGMA website:

Decision Pathways — Negotiating a Capitation Plan (case study)

Decision Pathways — Negotiating a Fee-for-Service Plan (case study)

Financial Management

Financial Management Tools

Medical Coding

Revenue Cycle Management

MGMA Connection Magazine — Financial Management Focus

Financial Management issue, published each February, is an array of articles that drill down into specific Body of Knowledge domain topics.

How to Get Paid is a special supplement.

Medical Practice Today, published each July, is a review of the annually updated "What Members Have to Say" research, focusing on challenges faced by MGMA members and what they're doing to survive and thrive in today's healthcare environment.

Payers & Providers: Finding Common Ground is a special supplement.

The State of Medical Practice, published each January, is an annual update to the myriad issues medical practice executives will grapple with in the coming year.

Version 5010 and the Future of Administrative Simplification is a special supplement.

MGMA Education — Conferences

Annual MGMA Financial Conference

Annual Medicare and Coding Update Webinars

MGMA Online Education — Self-Study Courses

Accounting Basics

Effective Debt Collection

Essentials of Financial Management

Financial Management Boot Camp

Financial Reporting and Analysis

Internal Control and Cash Flow

The Revenue Cycle

Index

Note: *ex.* indicates exhibit.

revenue recognition, 124-126
statements of income and retained
earnings, 127*ex.* *See also* Cash
flow statements
Advance Beneficiary Notice of Noncoverage
(ABN), 29
Allowables, 18
See also Contractual allowances
American Institute of Certified Public
Accountants (AICPA), 123
American Medical Association (AMA),
46
A/P. *See* Accounts payable (A/P)
A/R. *See* Accounts receivable (A/R)
Arbitration, 27
Assets, 115-117, 135-136, 190-192
See also Cash; Cash flow statements;
Chart of accounts; Investments;
Revenues
Association of Certified Fraud Examiners,
245, 253
Attestation, 236
Auditors
government, 241
independent (external), 241
internal, 241
See also CPAs (certified public
accountants)
Audits
adverse opinion, 240
coding, 2-3, 236-237
compliance, 234
disclaimer of opinion, 215
financial, 233-234, 235-236
key skills for management of, 233,
275
myth, 131
operational, 234
of payments, 25-27
qualified opinion, 238, 240
reports, 235, 238-240
revenue, 237
trail monitoring, 21

unqualified opinion, 238, 240*ex.*

Bankruptcy claims, 54
Benchmarks
A/R aging, 33-34
days in A/R, 31-33
external, 215-216
financial, 193-195
importance of, 41-42
internal, 215
MGMA Cost Survey, 30-32
MGMA Cost Survey examples,
218-219*ex.*, 220-221*ex.*, 222*ex.*,
224-225*ex.*
Billing
charge capture, 2, 4, 48
disputes, 48
by vendors, 81
See also Accounts receivable (A/R);
Collections
Billing staff functions
closing the books, 49
denial follow-up, 20
unpaid claim follow-up, 20-21
Bills. *See* Claims
Blue Cross Blue Shield, 5
Book value, 190
Break-even point, 195-196
Budgets
administrator duties, 165, 229-230
basics, 163
budgetary slack, 189
capital, 101-102, 104*ex.*, 167, 172,
170-171*ex.*
cash, 178-179, 186-187*ex.*
departmental, 179
depreciation, 190-192
expense, 172-173, 178-179*ex.*
and failure to allow enough time,
188
vs. financial accounting, 163-164
fixed vs. flexible, 186
master, 178, 182-183*ex.*, 184-185*ex.*
methodologies, 186-188

System (HCPCS), 3, 46
Healthcare Effectiveness Data and Information Set (HEDIS), 16, 44
High-deductible insurance plans, 10, 18

Income tax basis statements, 123-124, 119*ex.*
Indemnification, 62
Indemnity policies, 10
Indirect costs, 199-200
Insurance
  dishonesty, 251
  health, 5-6, 10
  noncoverage situations, 29-30
  primary, 22
  private, 43
  secondary, 22
  workers' compensation, 9-10
  see also Payers
Insurance companies, 5, 43
Internal cash controls
  bank reconciliation, 147, 273, 274*ex.*
  cash disbursements, 260-265, 260*ex.*
  cash receipts, 258-260, 259*ex.*
  checklist, 271, 272*ex.*
  communication, 265-266
  control activities, 256-265
  control self-assessment (CSA), 267
  cost-effectiveness, 258
  credit card access, 263
  detective, 257
  electronic payments, 262
  employee screening and training, 253
  ethics training, 254
  evaluations, 267-268
  facsimile signature stamps, 149, 262
  general, 253
  information system, 257
  internet banking, 273-275
  monitoring, 266-267
  physical, 257

policies and procedures, 256
preventive, 257
purpose of, 107, 253
risk assessment, 255
segregation of duties, 148-149, 254, 255*ex.*, 258-262, 259*ex.*
Internal collections, 30, 52-57
Internal Revenue Code, 159
International Classification of Diseases, 10th revision, Clinical Modification (ICD-10-CM), 3, 45-46
Investing activities, 88, 88*ex.*, 101, 108-110
Investments
  forecasting capital needs, 206-211
  long-range, 201
  managing, 200-211
  managing short-term, 108-110
  nonfinancial performance measures, 205-206
  proposals, 183-184
  short-range, 201-202

  time value of money, 202
  utilization analysis, 204

Joint Commission, The, 44
Journals, 142-145

Liabilities, 135-135
Liquid-asset funds, 109
Liquidity, 86
Litigation, 27
Loans. *See* Financing activities

Mackay, Harvey, 81
Managed care
  and capitation, 14, 82
  health maintenance organizations (HMOs), 7
  overview, 6-7
  preferred provider organizations (PPOs), 7, 13
Management accounting, 192

estimates of, 131
formula for total medical, 37
net vs. gross, 42
projected cash receipts, 98-99,
101*ex.*
recognition of in accounting methods, 124-126
Risk
in contracts, 61-64
financial, 15, 85
and financial flexibility, 86
forecasting capital needs, 206-211
and global capitation, 14
operating, 85-86
See also Fraud and theft; Internal
cash controls

Savings accounts, 109
Scope paragraph, 238
Section 179 deduction, 191
Segregation of duties, 148-149, 254,
258-262, 255*ex.*, 259*ex.*, 260*ex.*
Self-payer, 7-8, 55
Short-term borrowing, 104-105
Short-term investments, 108-110
Silent preferred provider organizations
(PPOs), 13
Small claims court, 54-55
Stakeholders
explaining financial information to,
222
one-on-one discussions with, 228
oral presentations to, 226-227
providing financial information to,
217
technological communication with,
228-229
visual communication to, 228
written communication to, 223, 226
State Children's Health Insurance Program, 36
Statement of financial position, 135-136
Steerage, 11
Step-fixed cost, 195

Strategic planning, 164
*Swim with the Sharks without Being Eaten
Alive*, 81

Tax basis statements, 124, 128*ex.*
Tax Equity and Fiscal Responsibility Act
(1982), 9
Taxes
CPA services for, 243-244
deferred, 126, 130, 131-132
depreciation, 191-192
Federal Unemployment Tax Act,
158
federal withholding, 156
local, 158
Medicare, 157
payroll, 156-159
Section 179 deduction, 191
Social Security, 156-157
state unemployment insurance, 158
state withholding, 157
Theft. *See* Fraud and theft
Third-party payers, 3, 16-18, 24*ex.*
Time value of money, 202
Transactions, 142-143
TRICARE, 9
*2012 Report to the Nations on Occupation-
al Fraud and Abuse*, 254

Uninsured patients, 6
U.S. Department of Health and Human
Services, Office of Inspector General,
255
U.S. Treasury bills, 109
Utilization analysis, 204

Variable costs, 193, 1954
Vendors, payments to, 81
See also Accounts payable (A/P)

Welch, Jack, 189
Withhold tracking, 21
Workers' Compensation, 9
Write-offs, 56-57
See also Contractual allowances

CPSIA information can be obtained
at www.ICGtesting.com
Printed in the USA
FSHW021811151219
64846FS

9 781568 296937